Bondage Coloring Book

55 Beautiful BDSM Scenes for Adult Coloring

Felice Lammermoore

The author would like to extend a heart felt thank you to Heather aka Secretsxywriter from Literotica for her valuable feedback and input during the creation of this project.

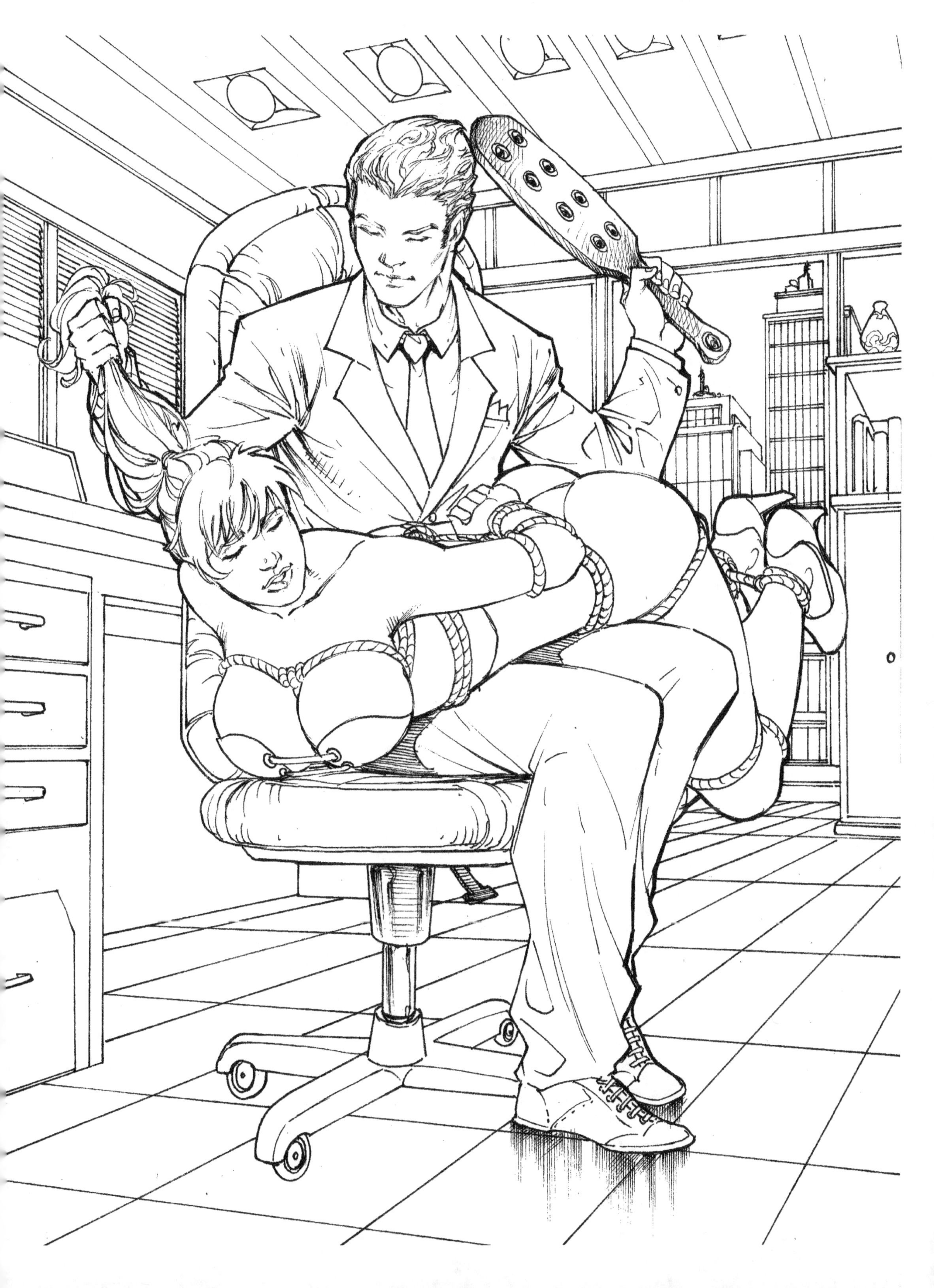

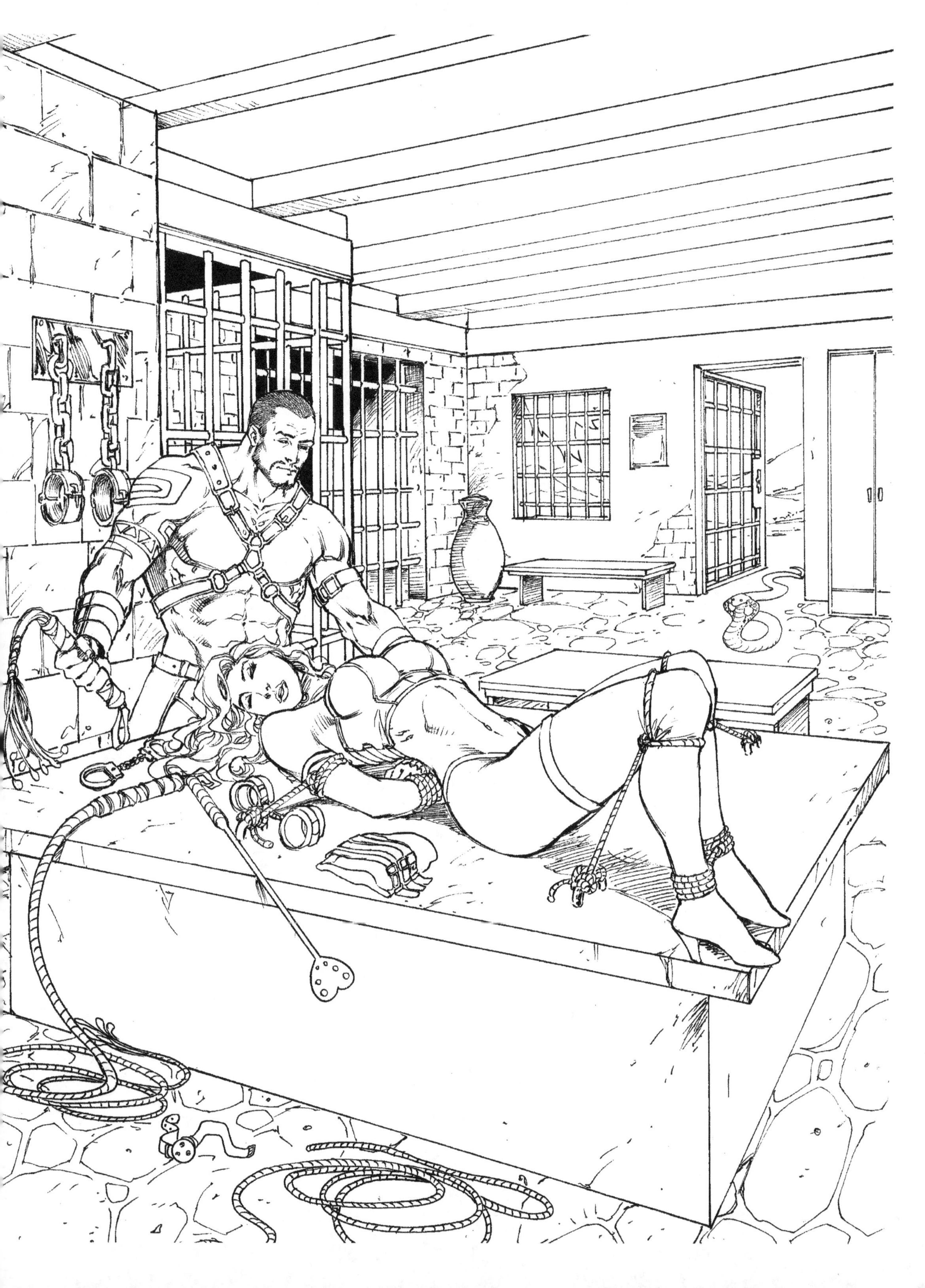

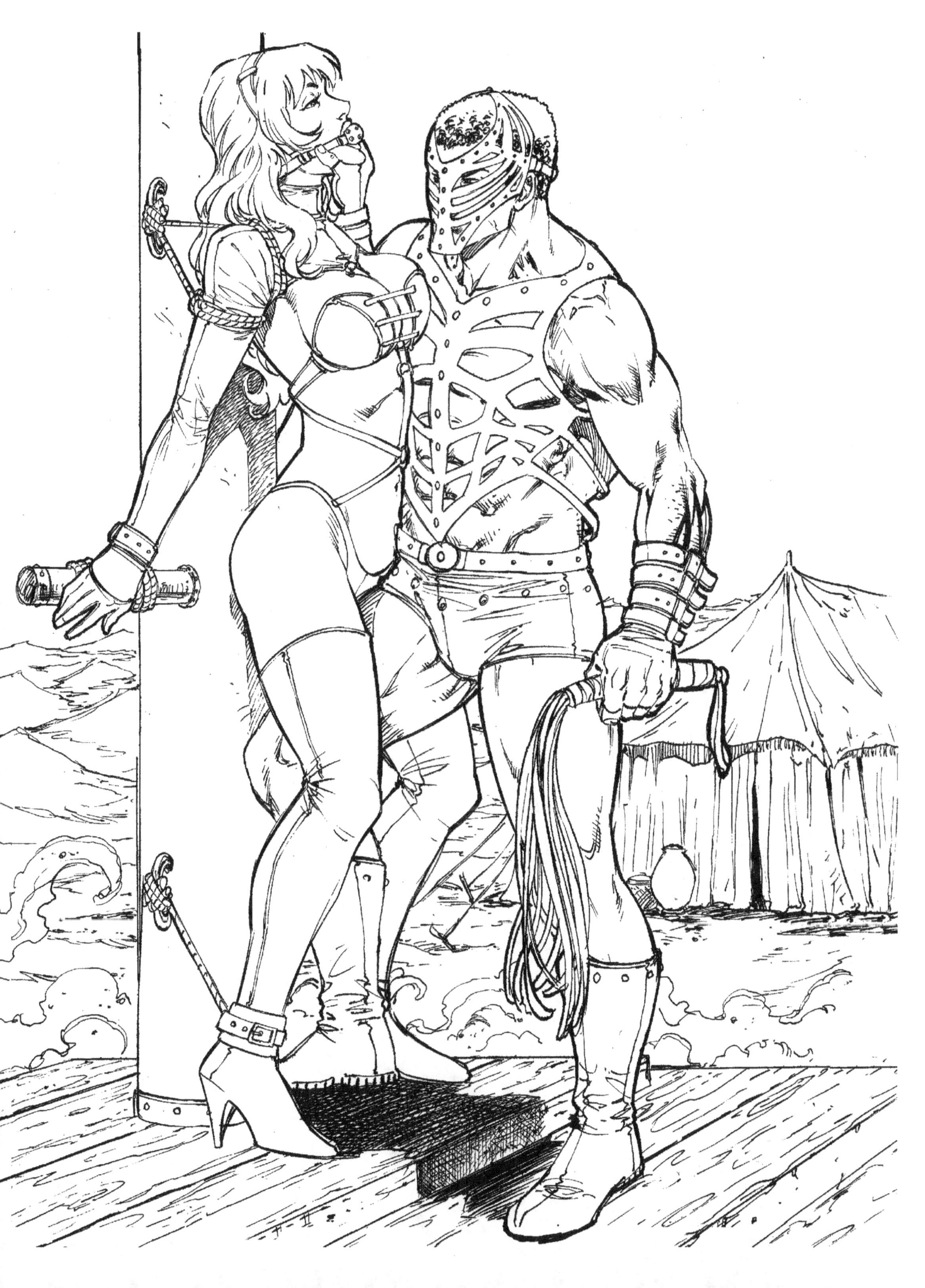

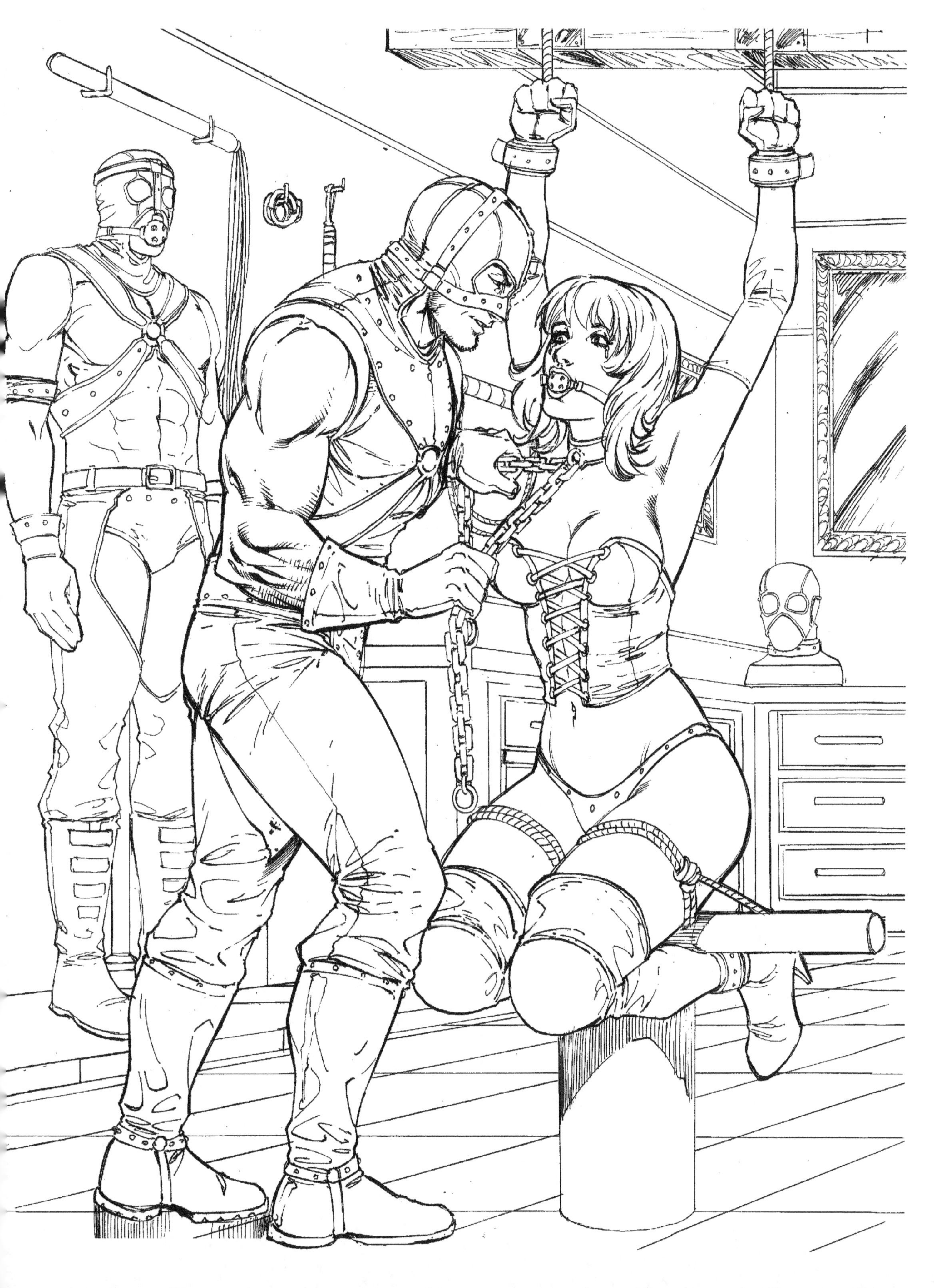

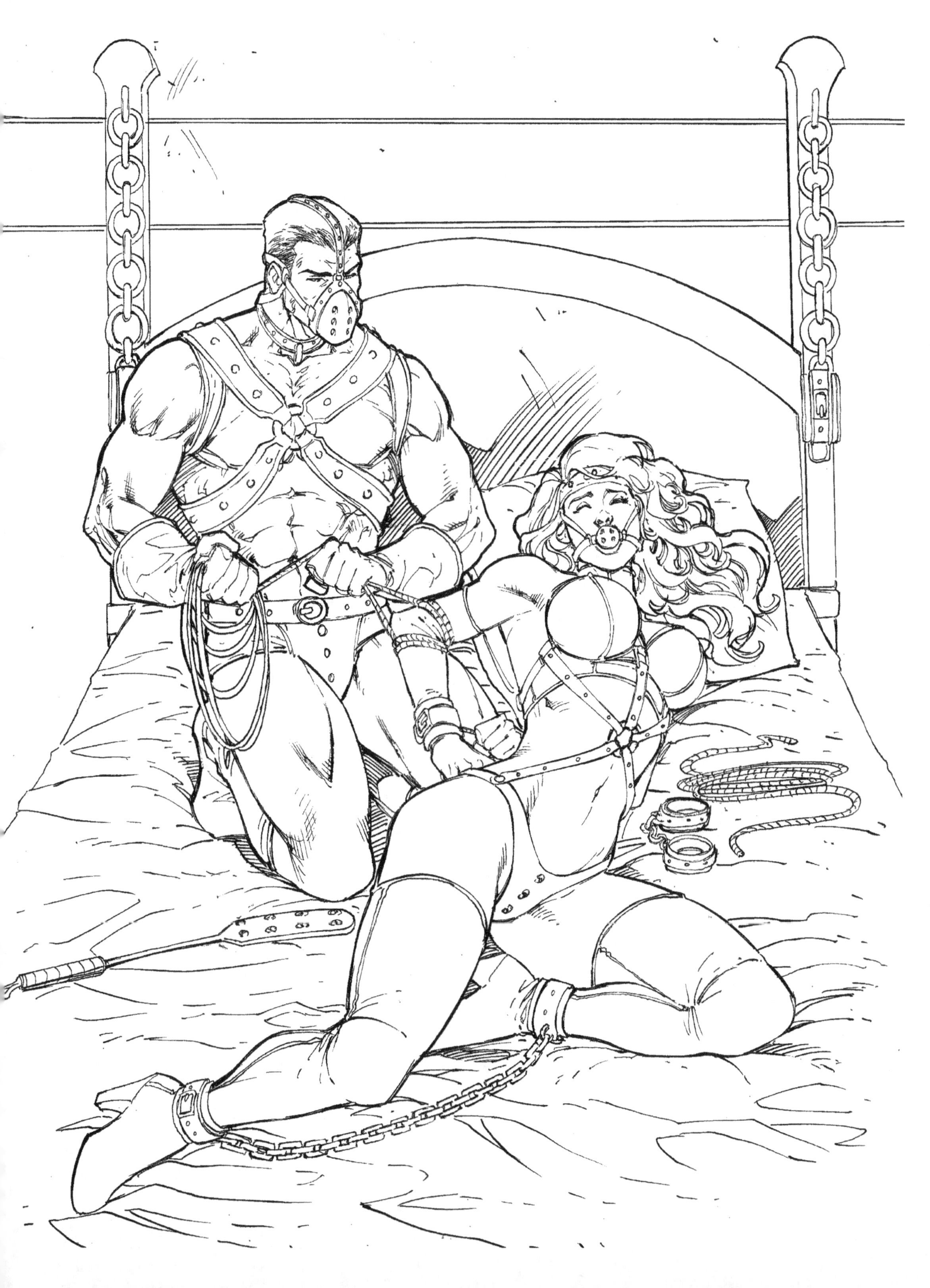

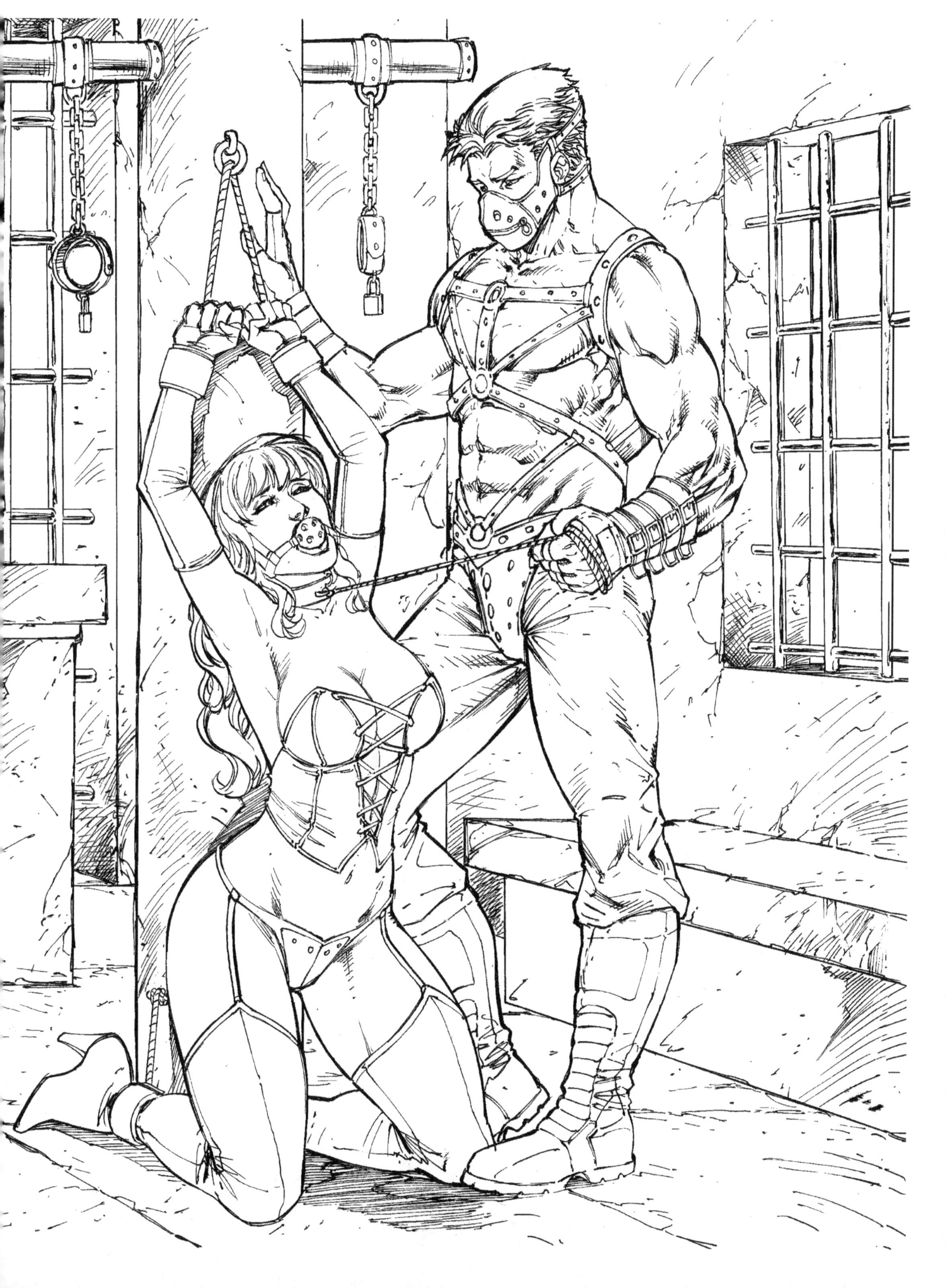

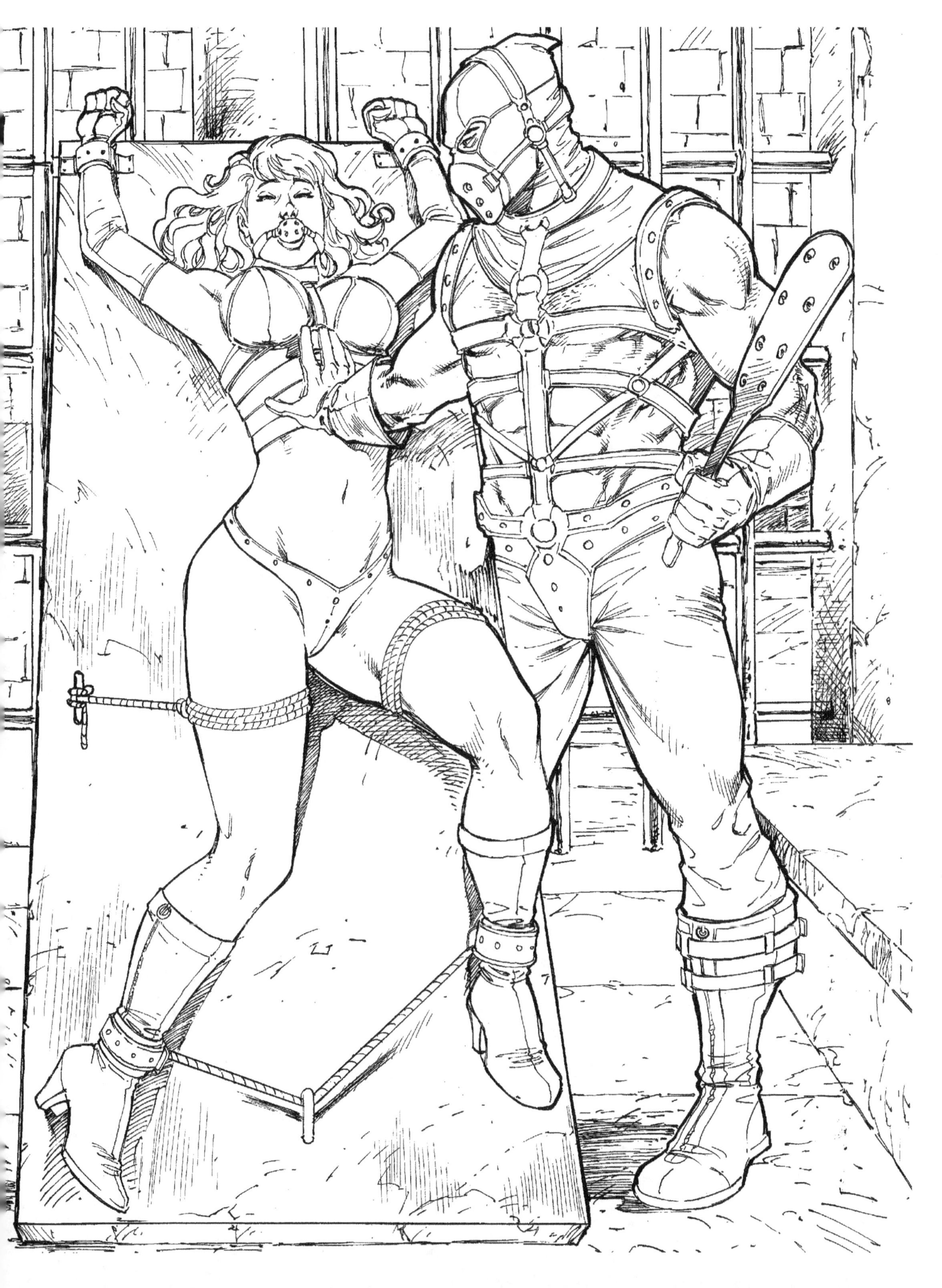

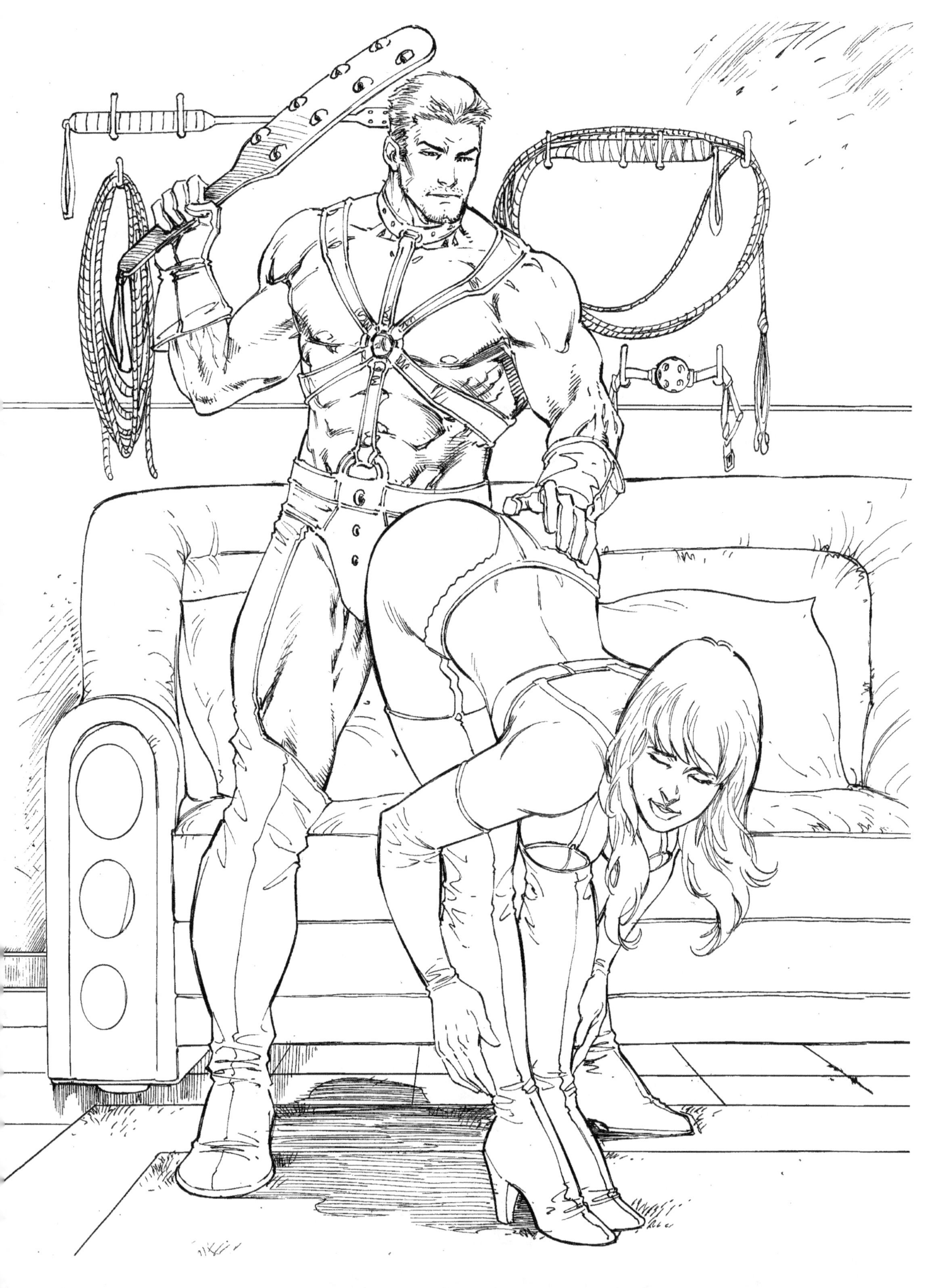

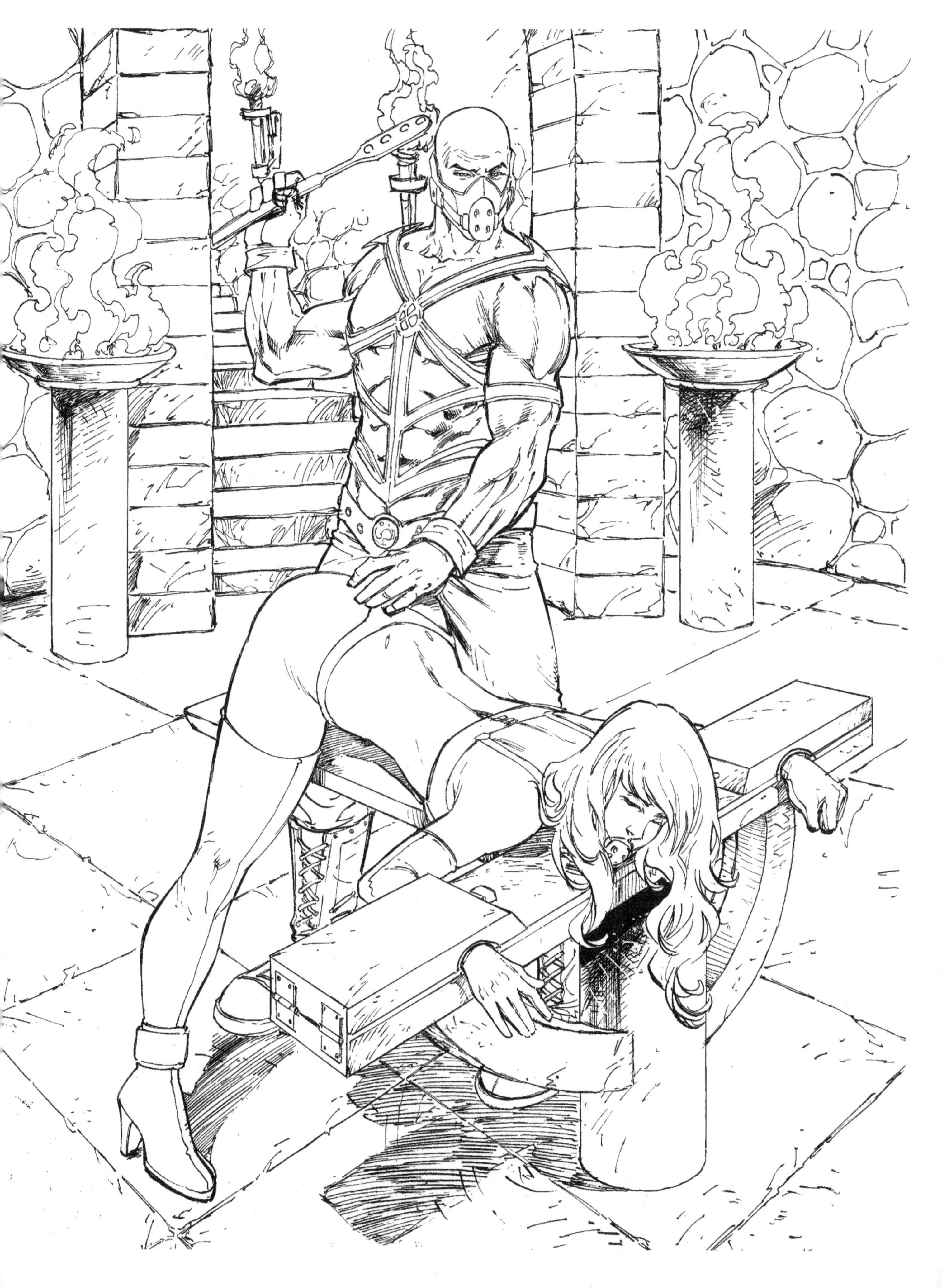

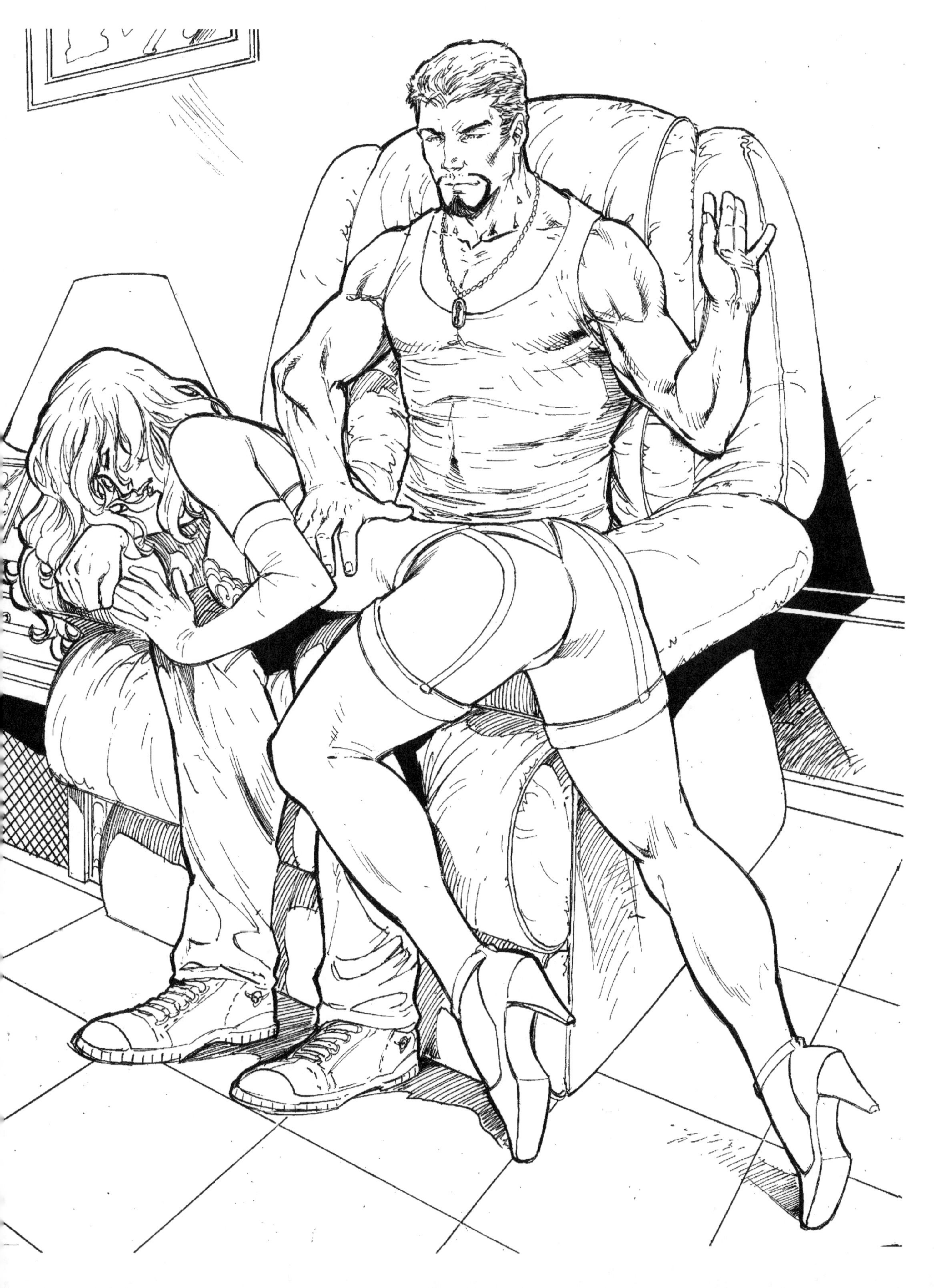

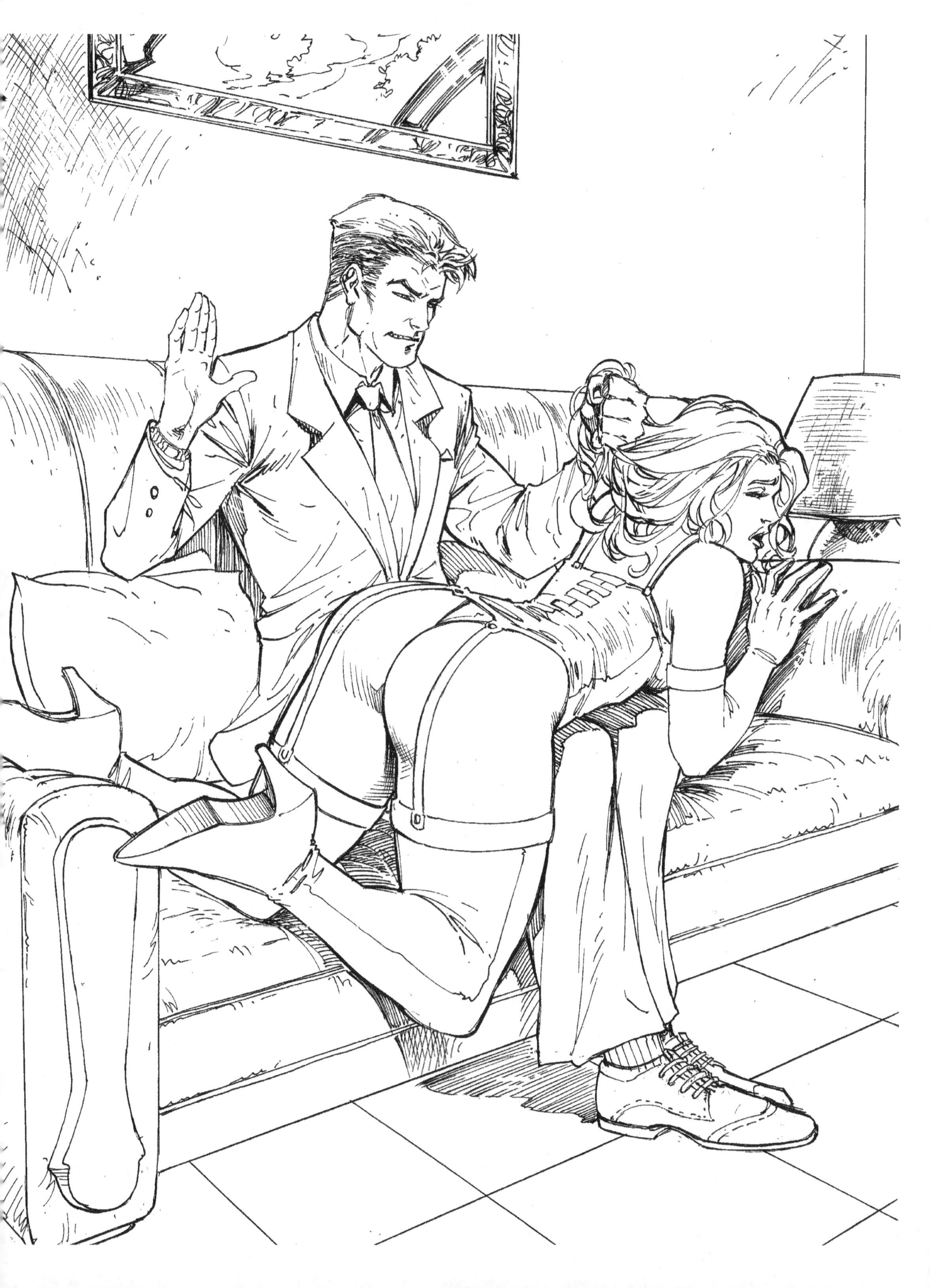

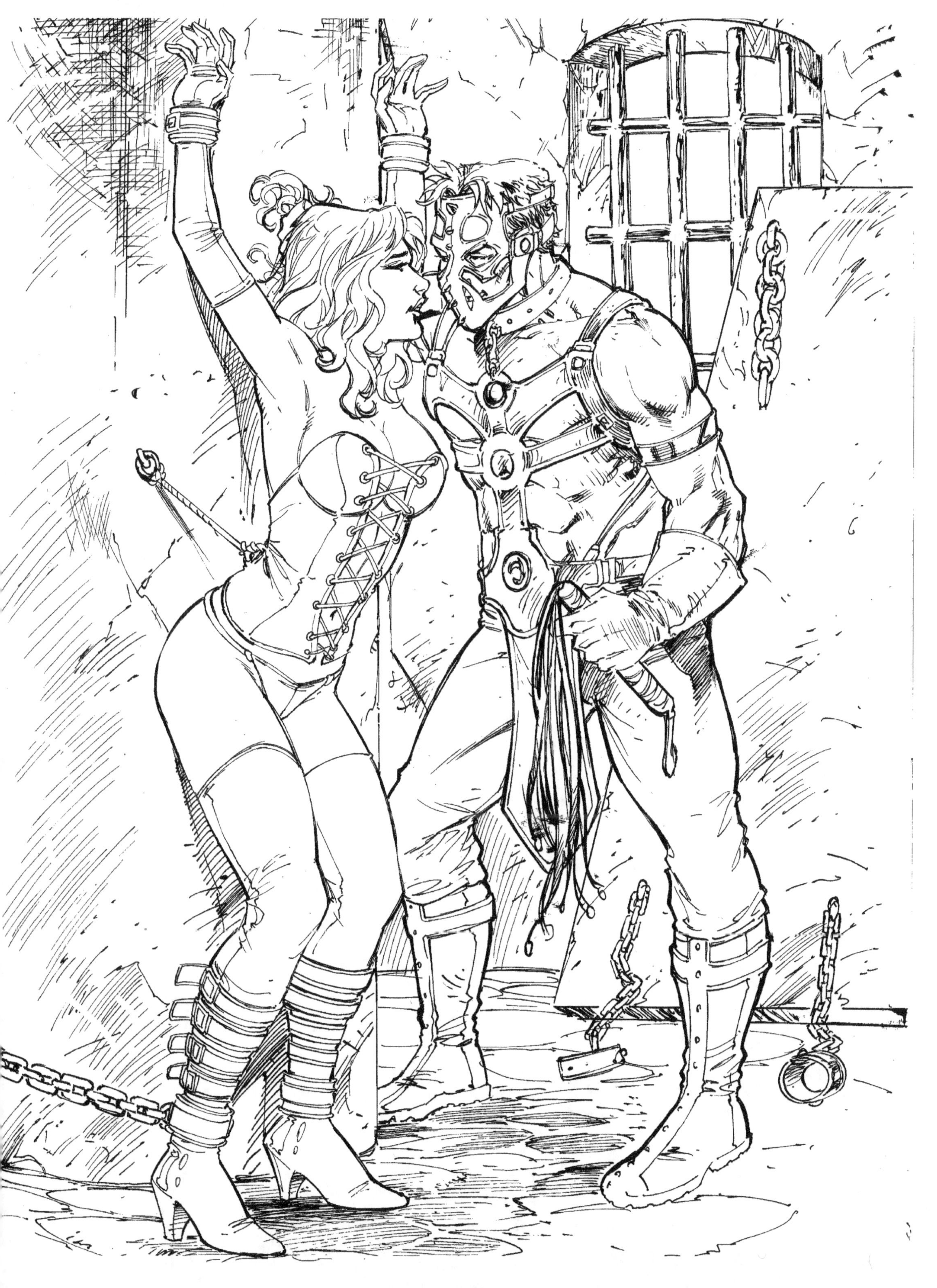

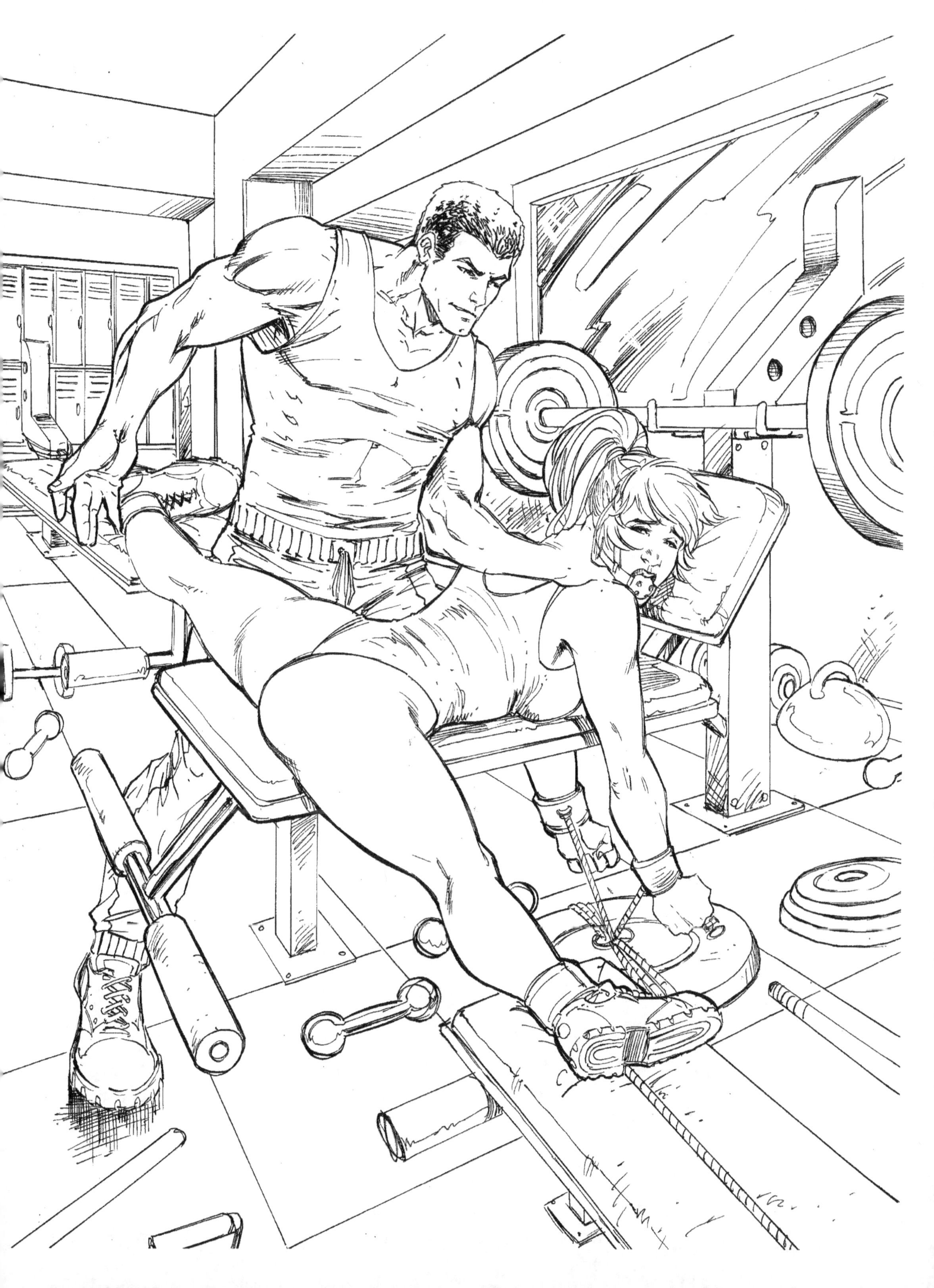

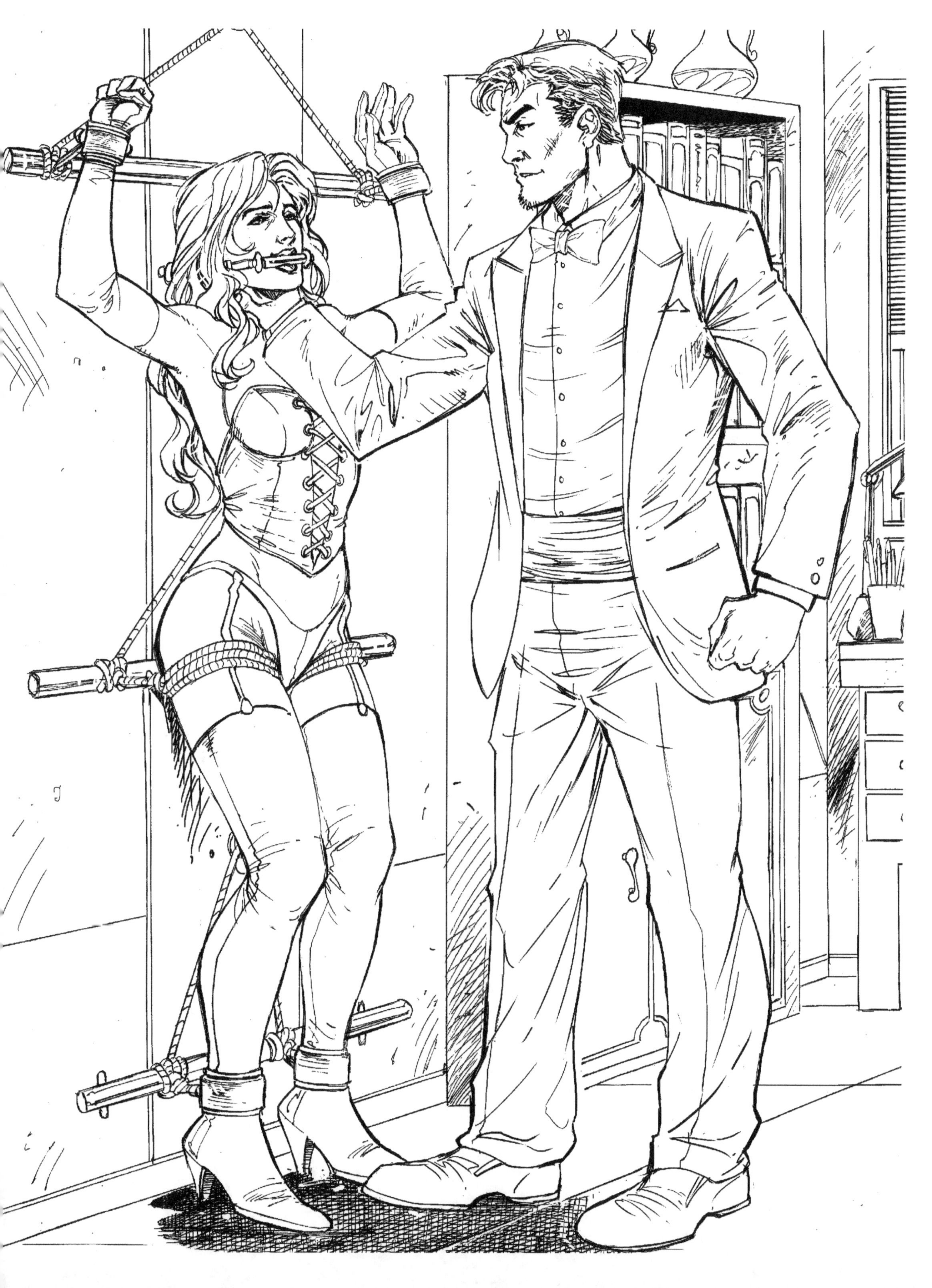

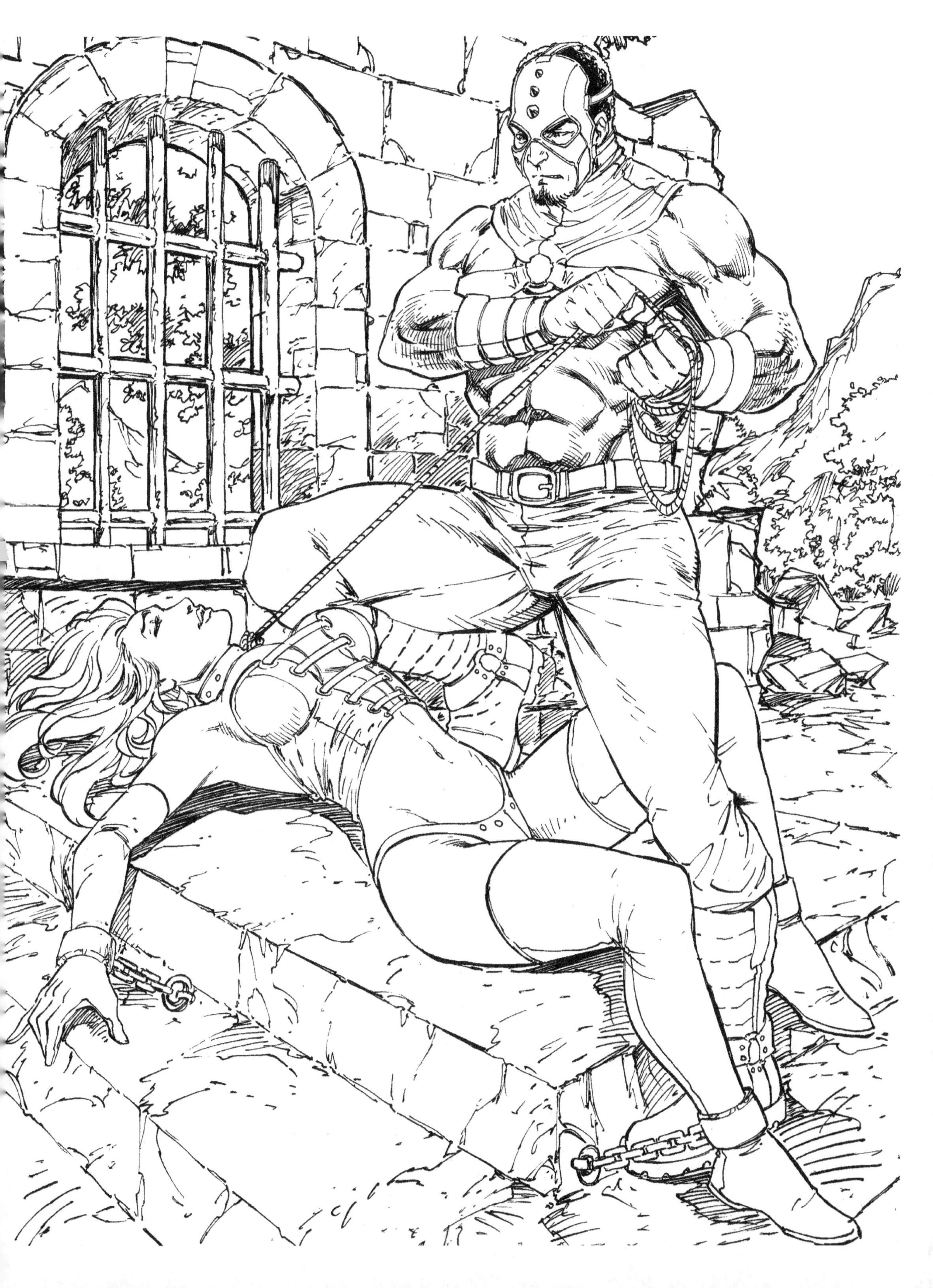

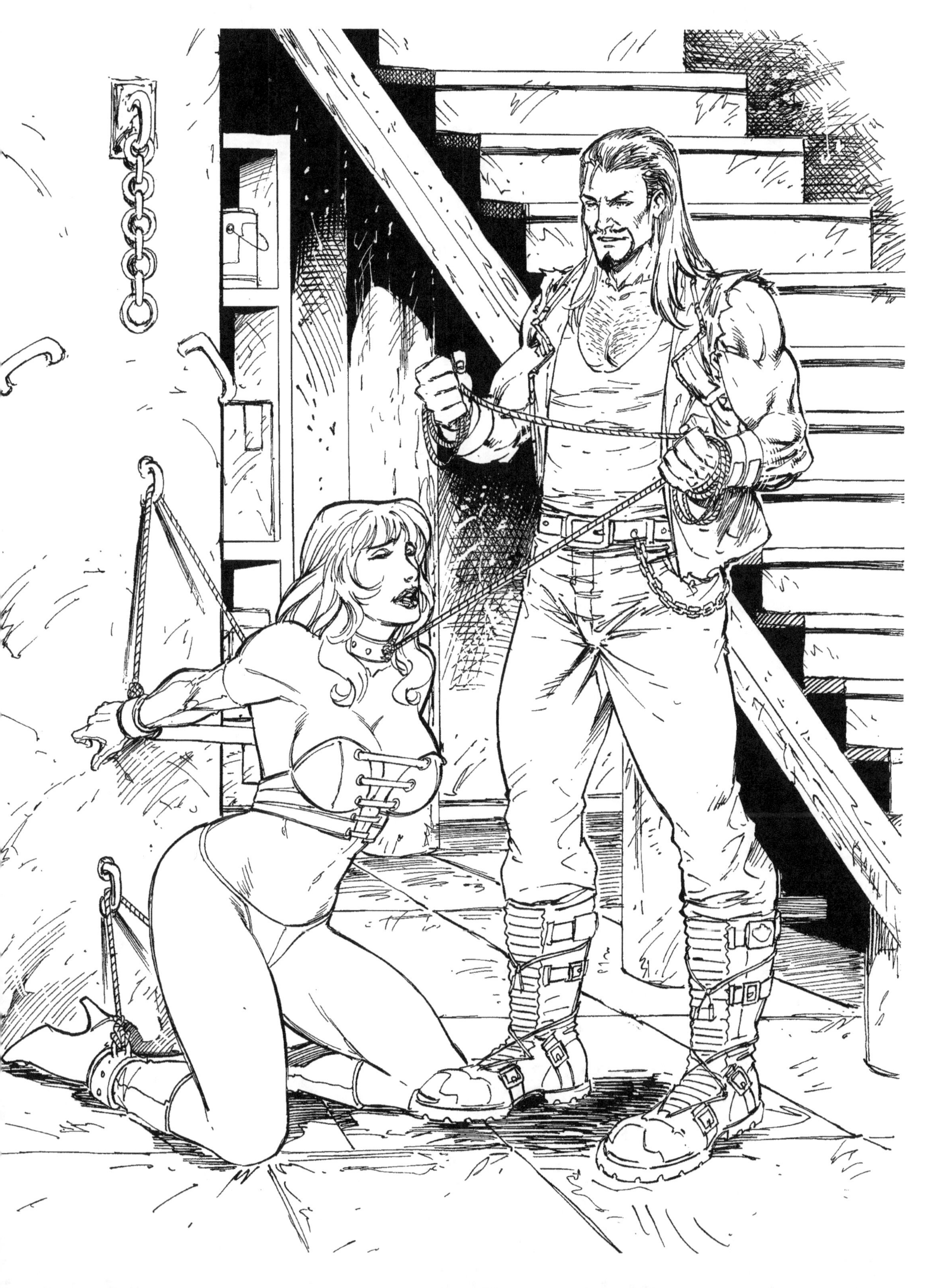

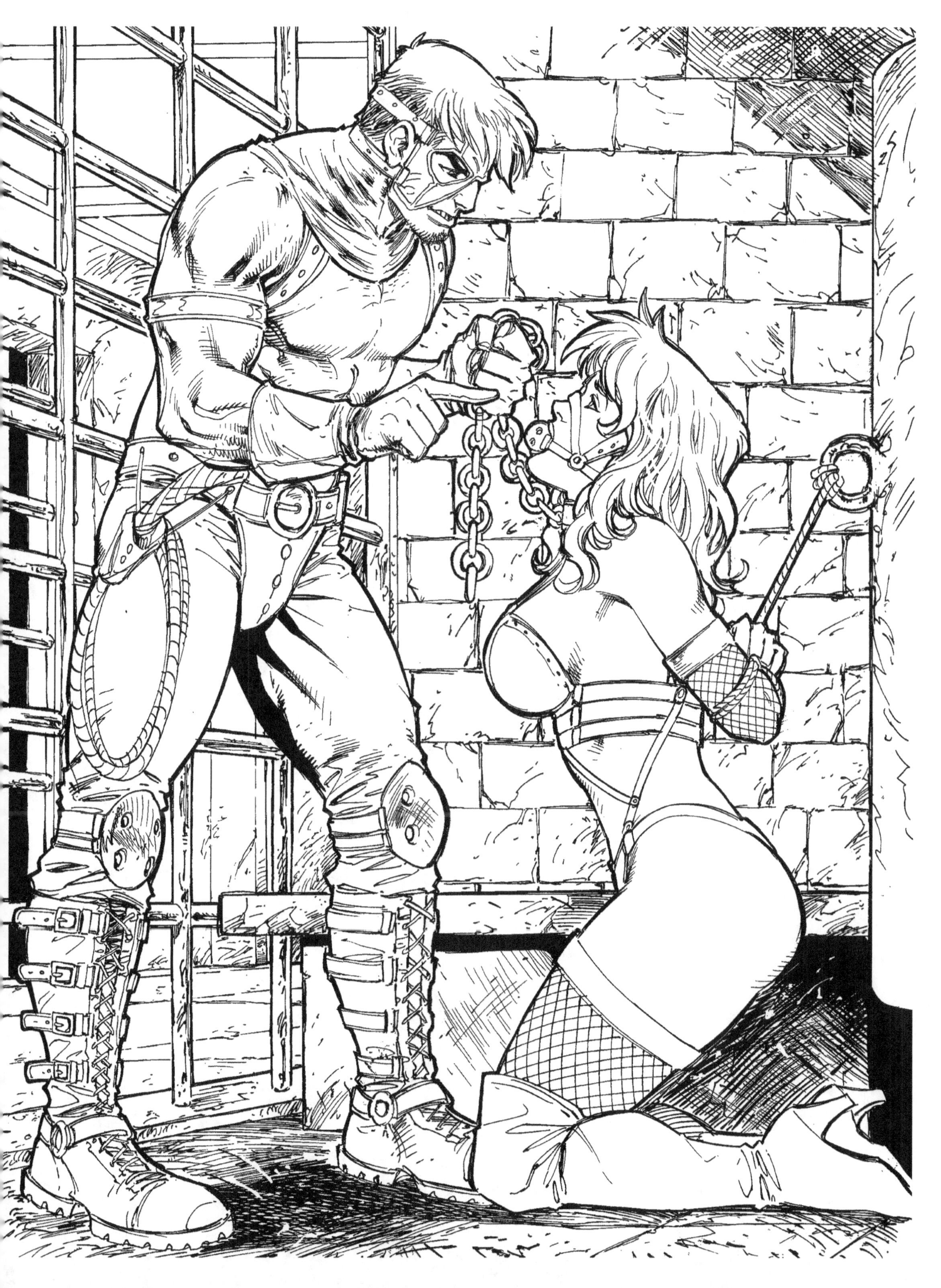

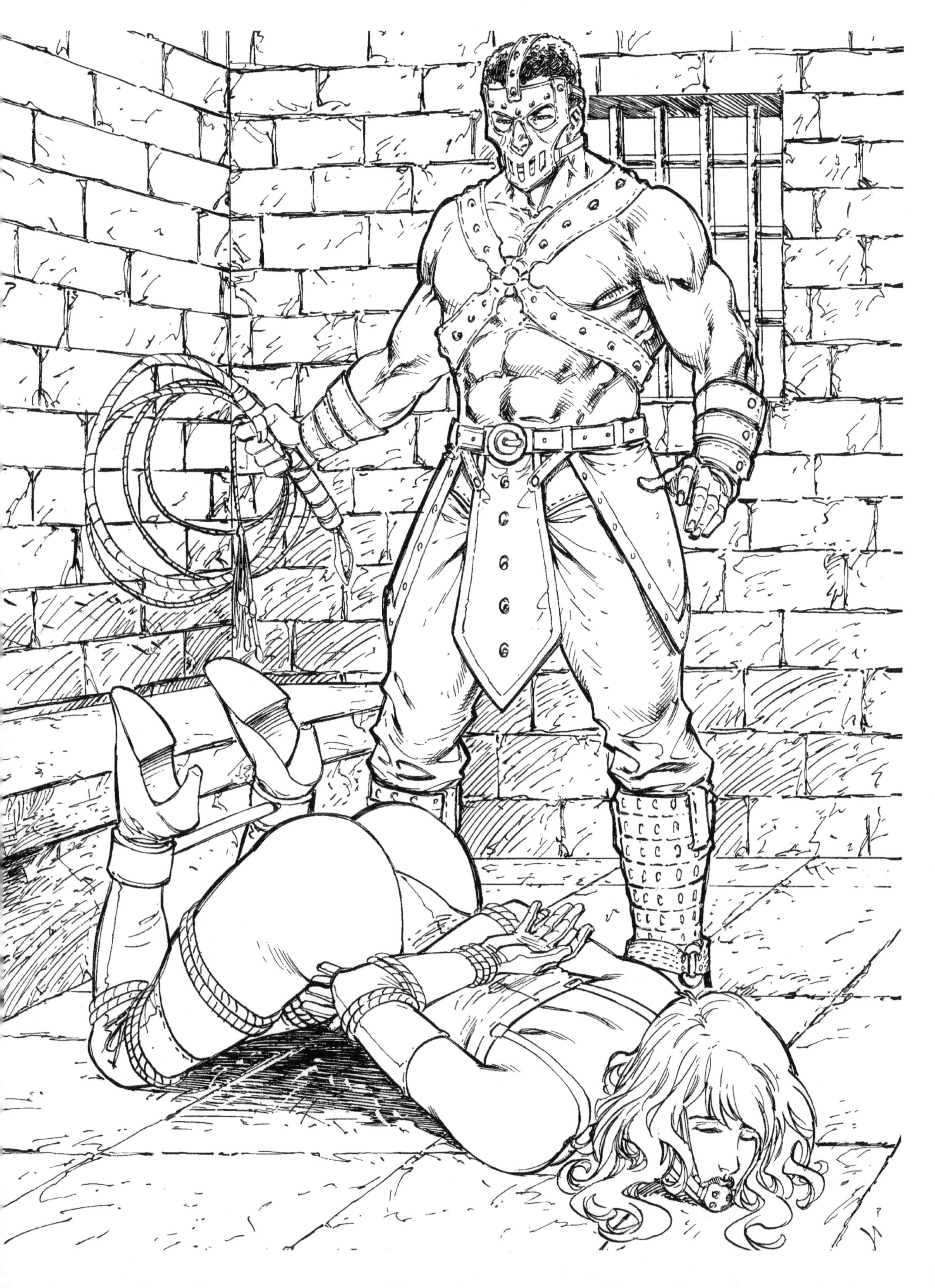

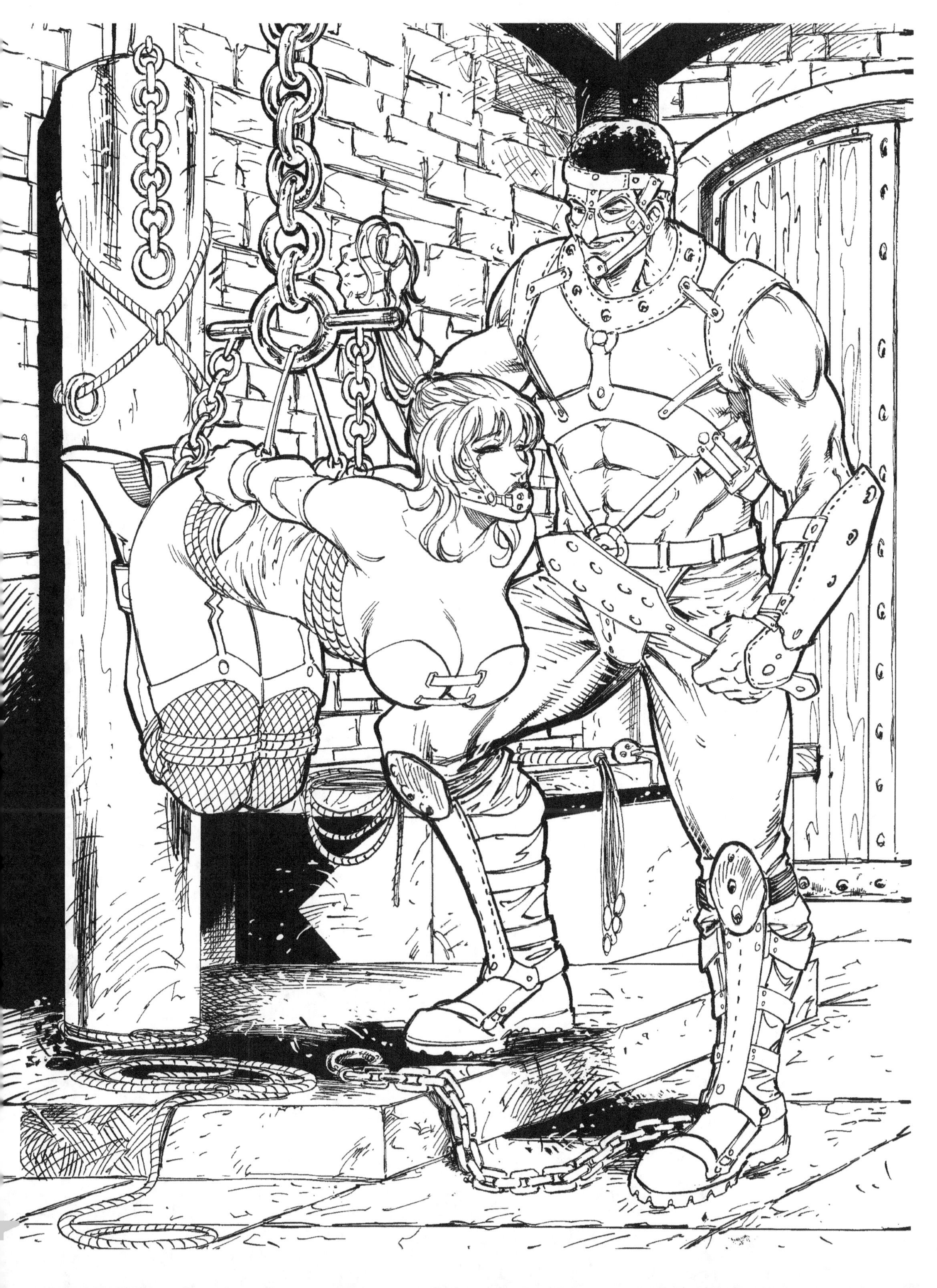

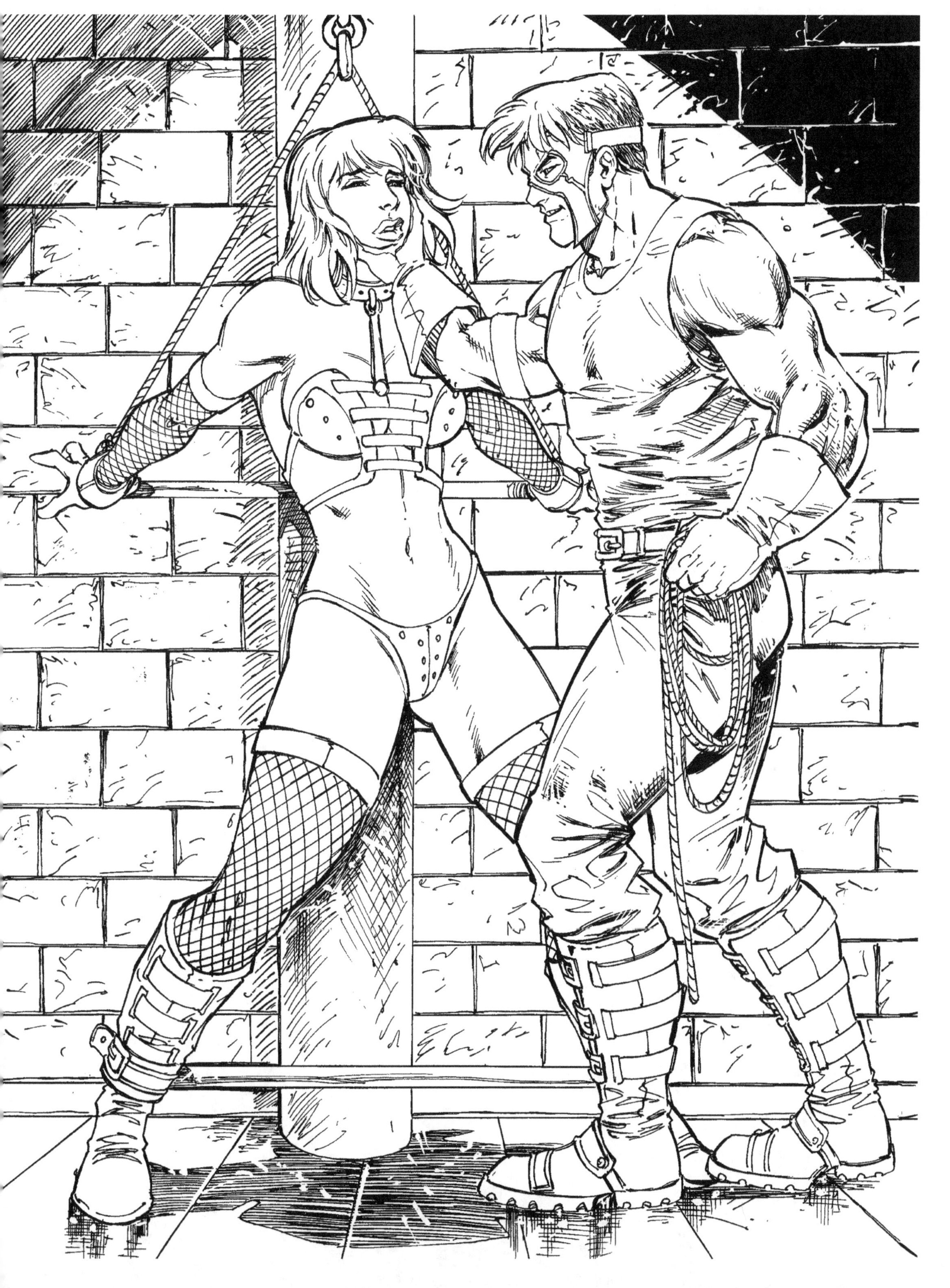

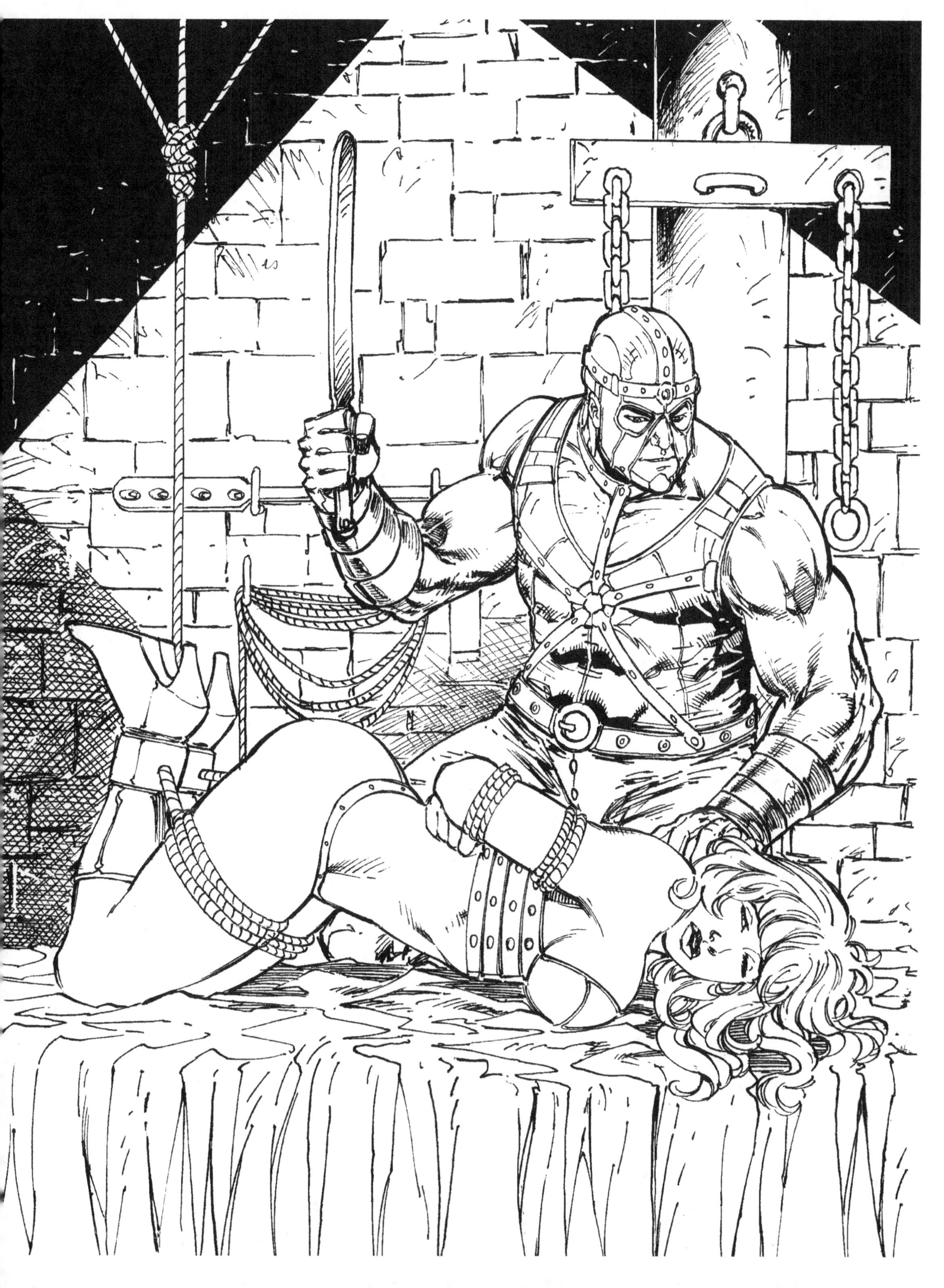

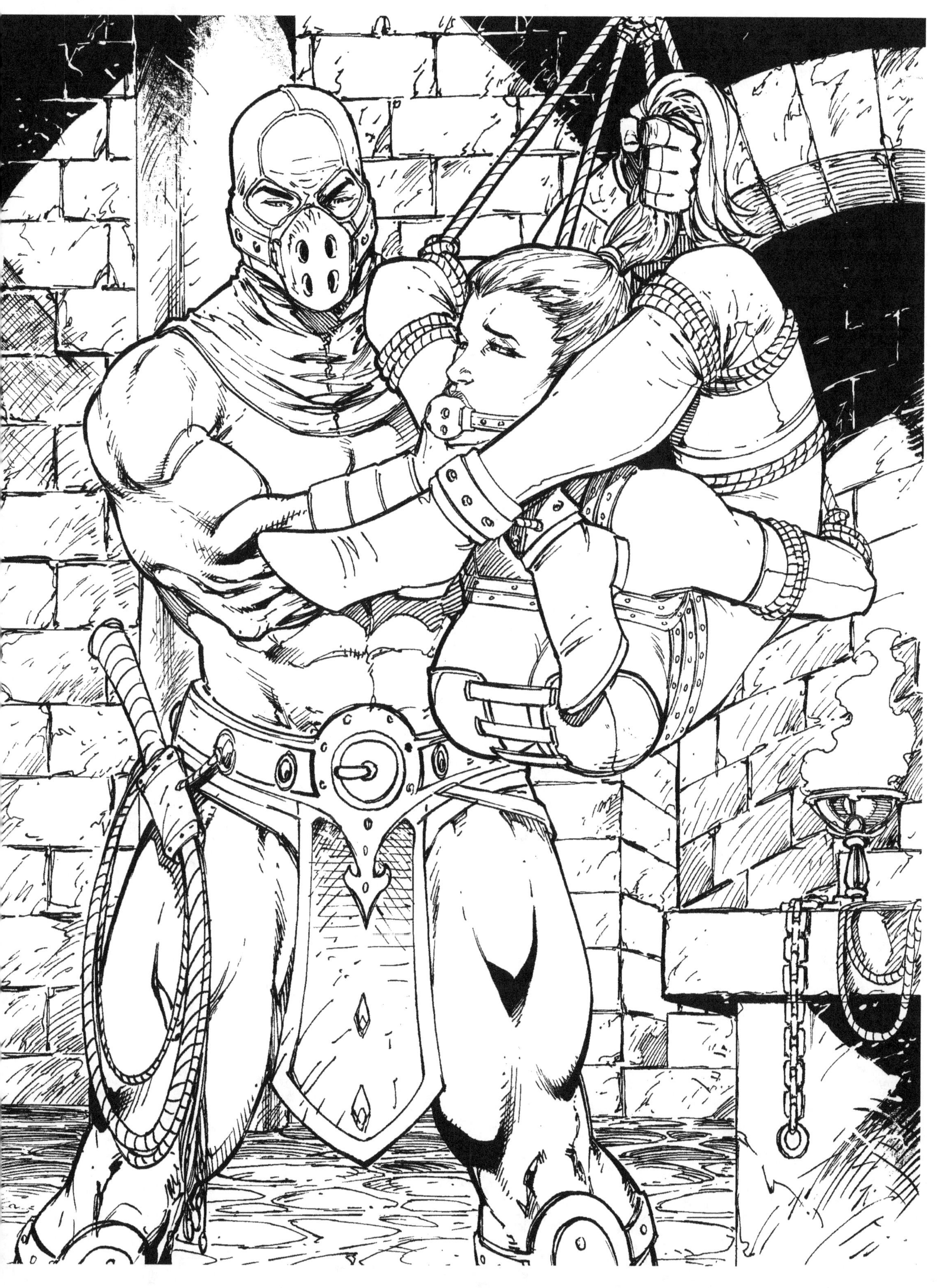

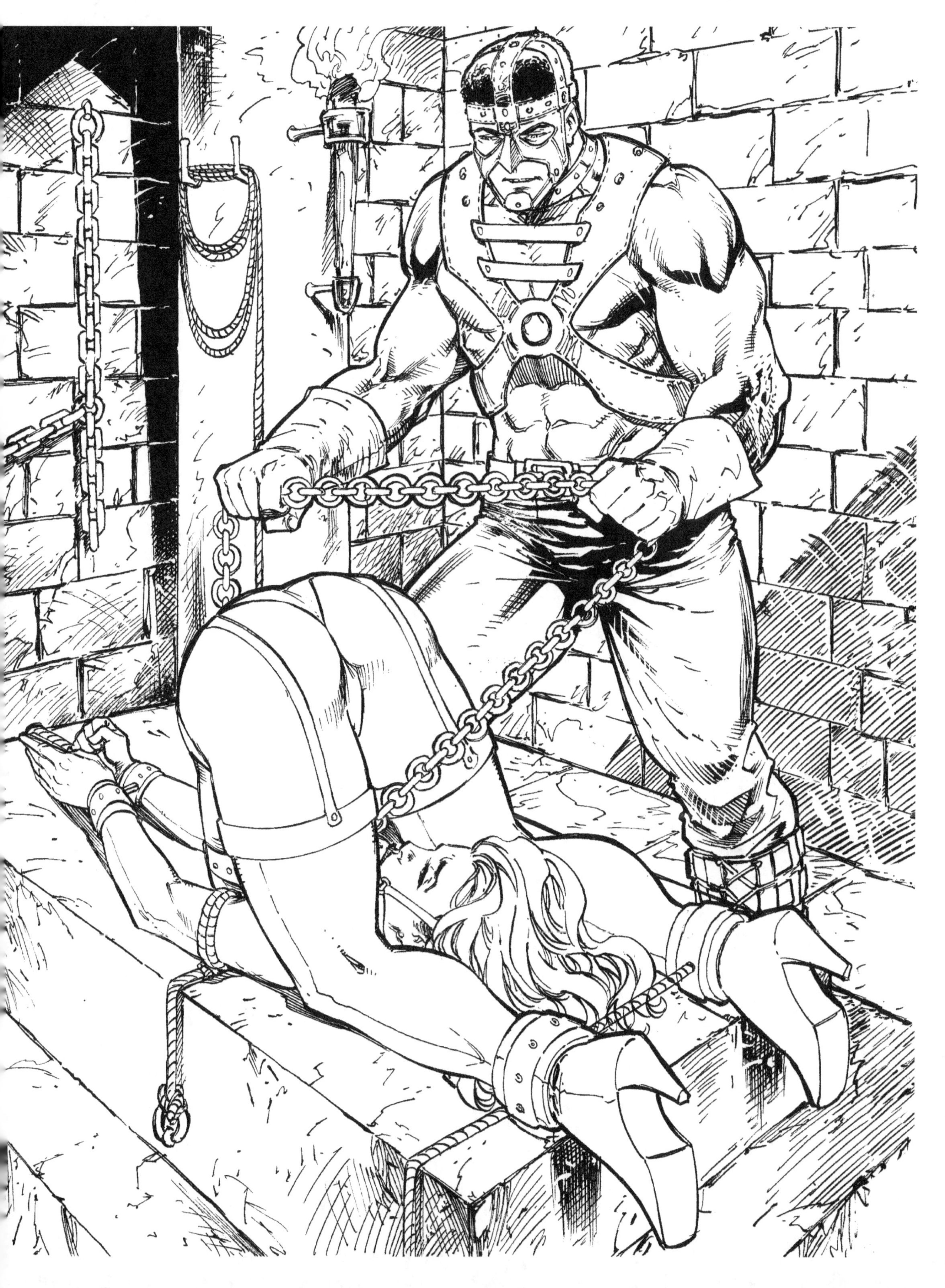

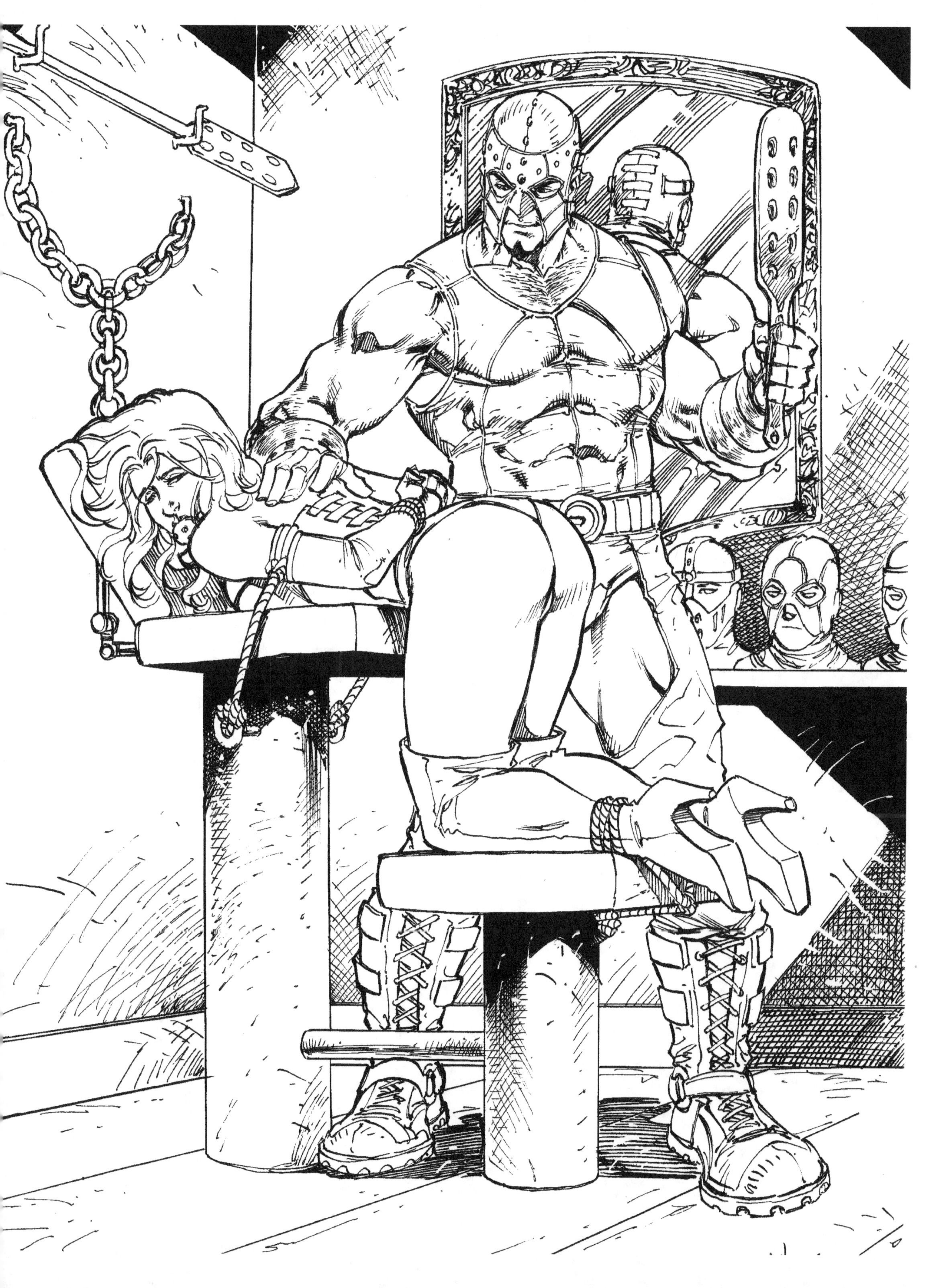

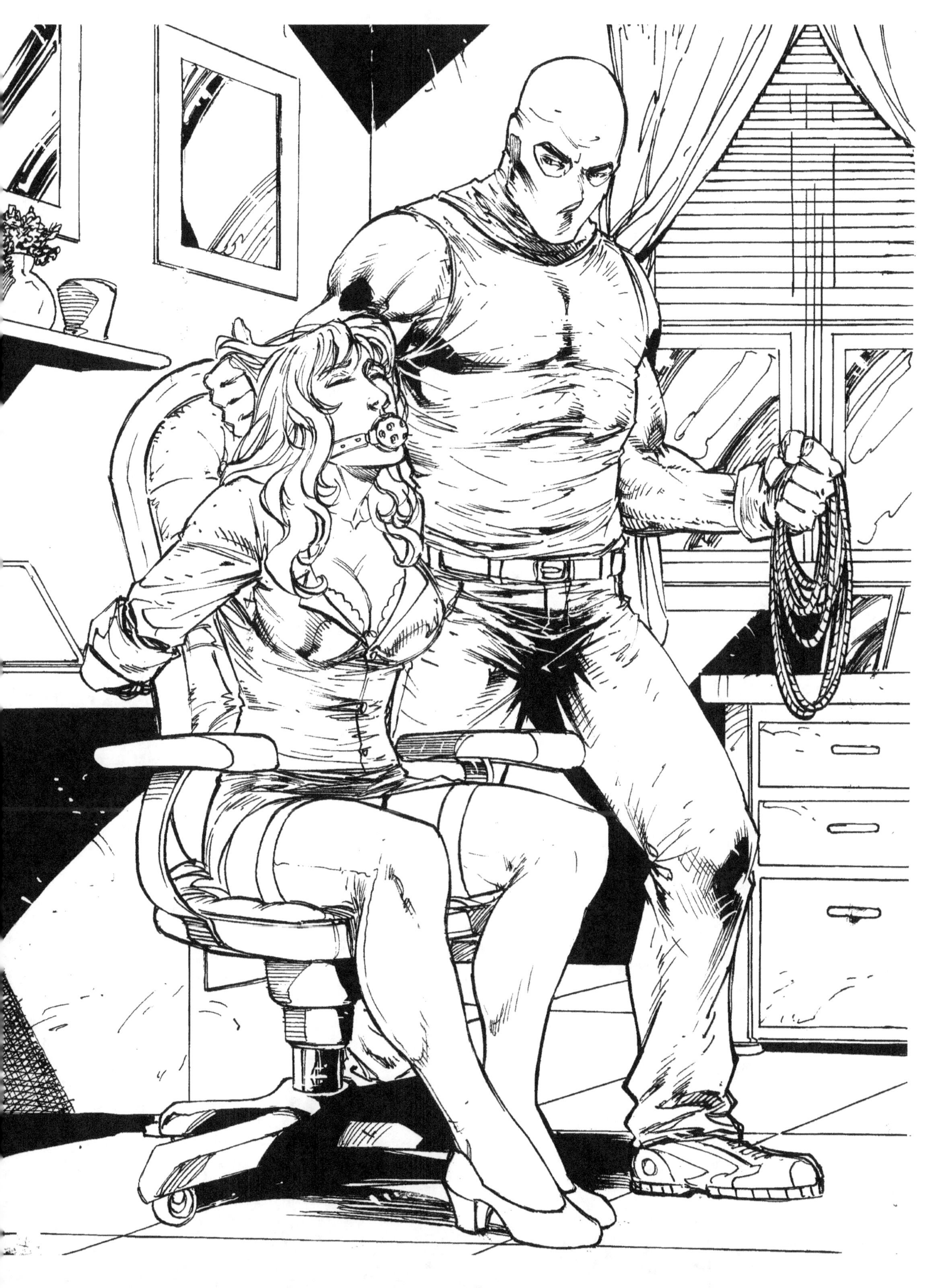

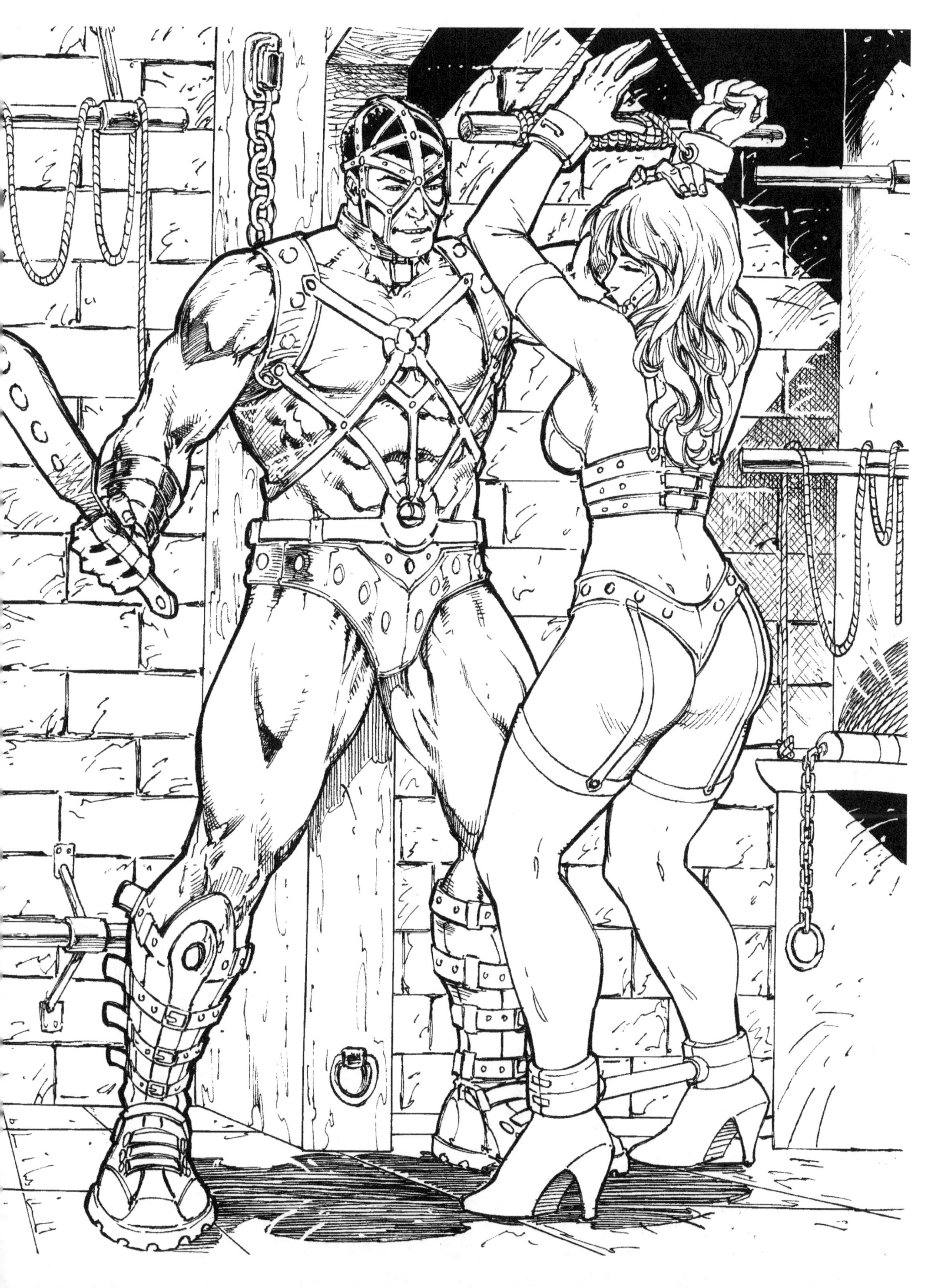

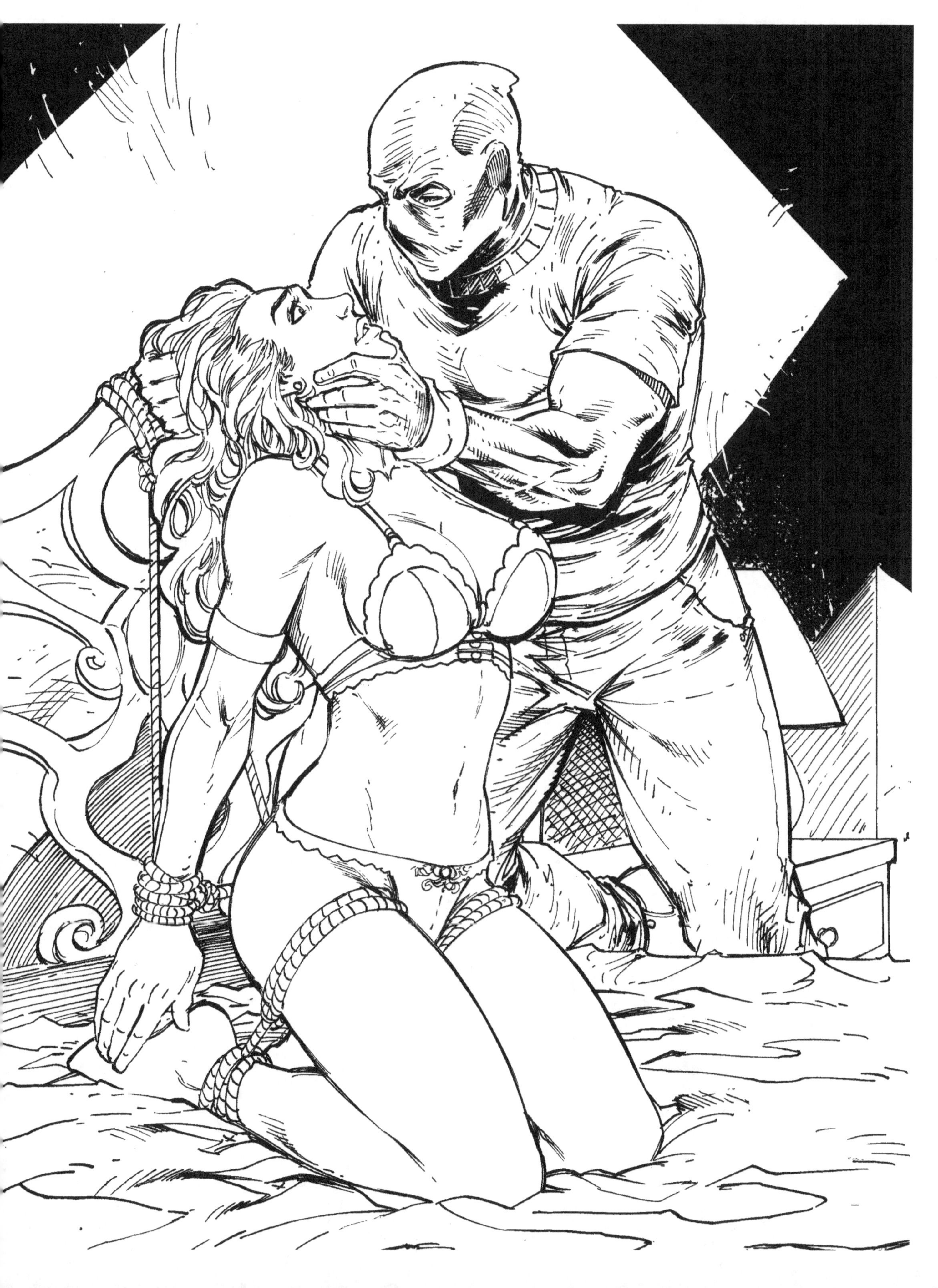

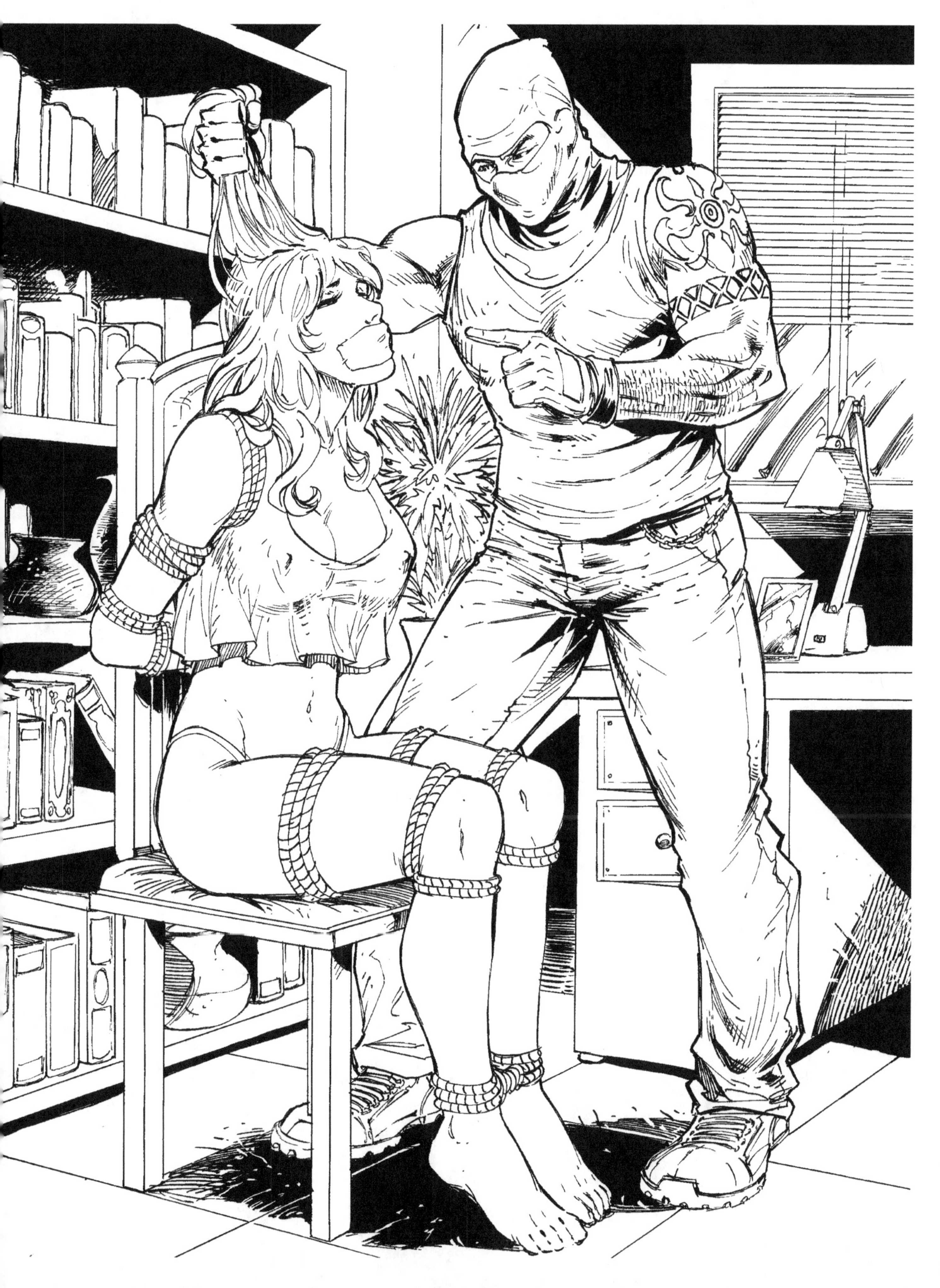

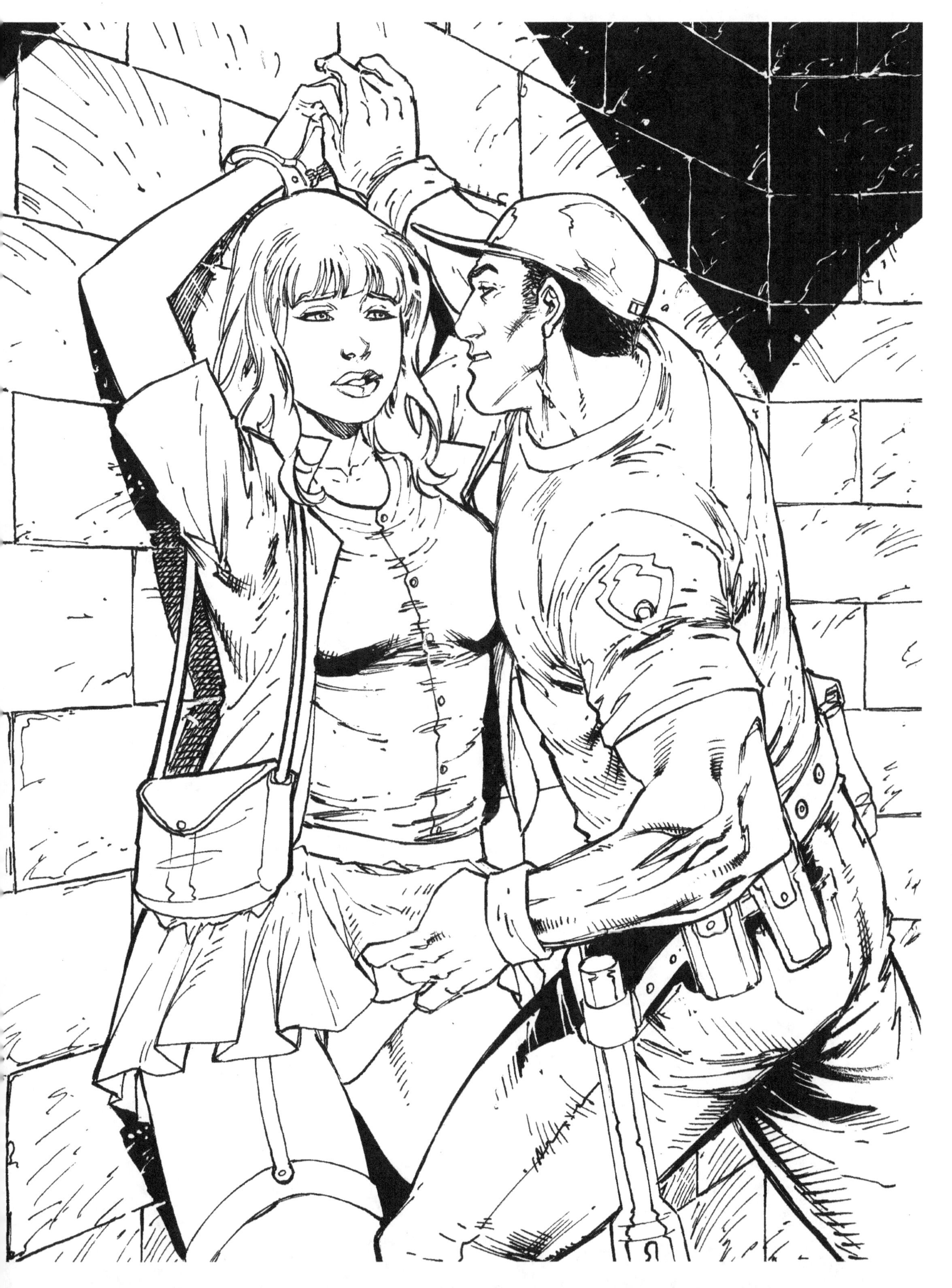

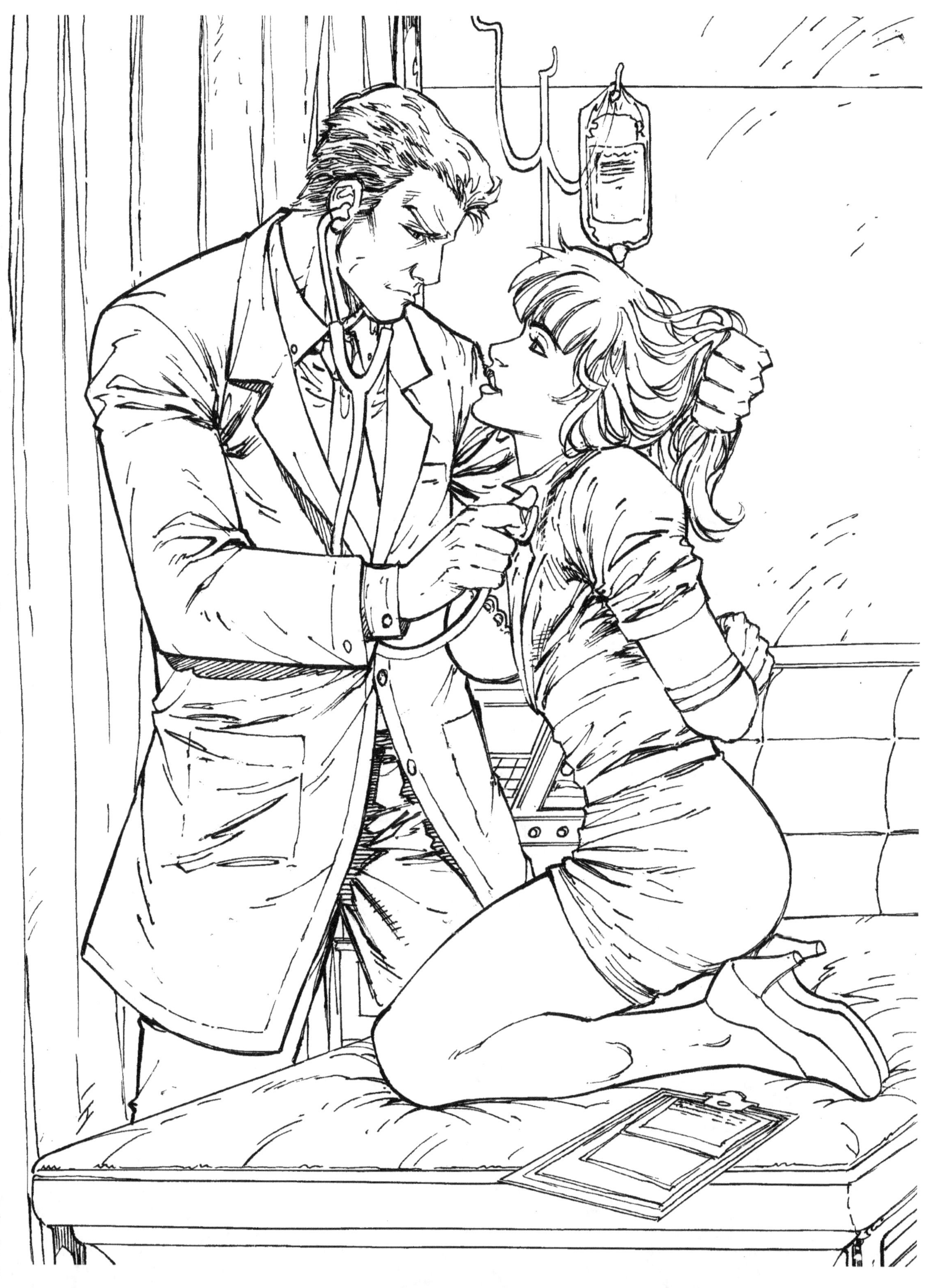

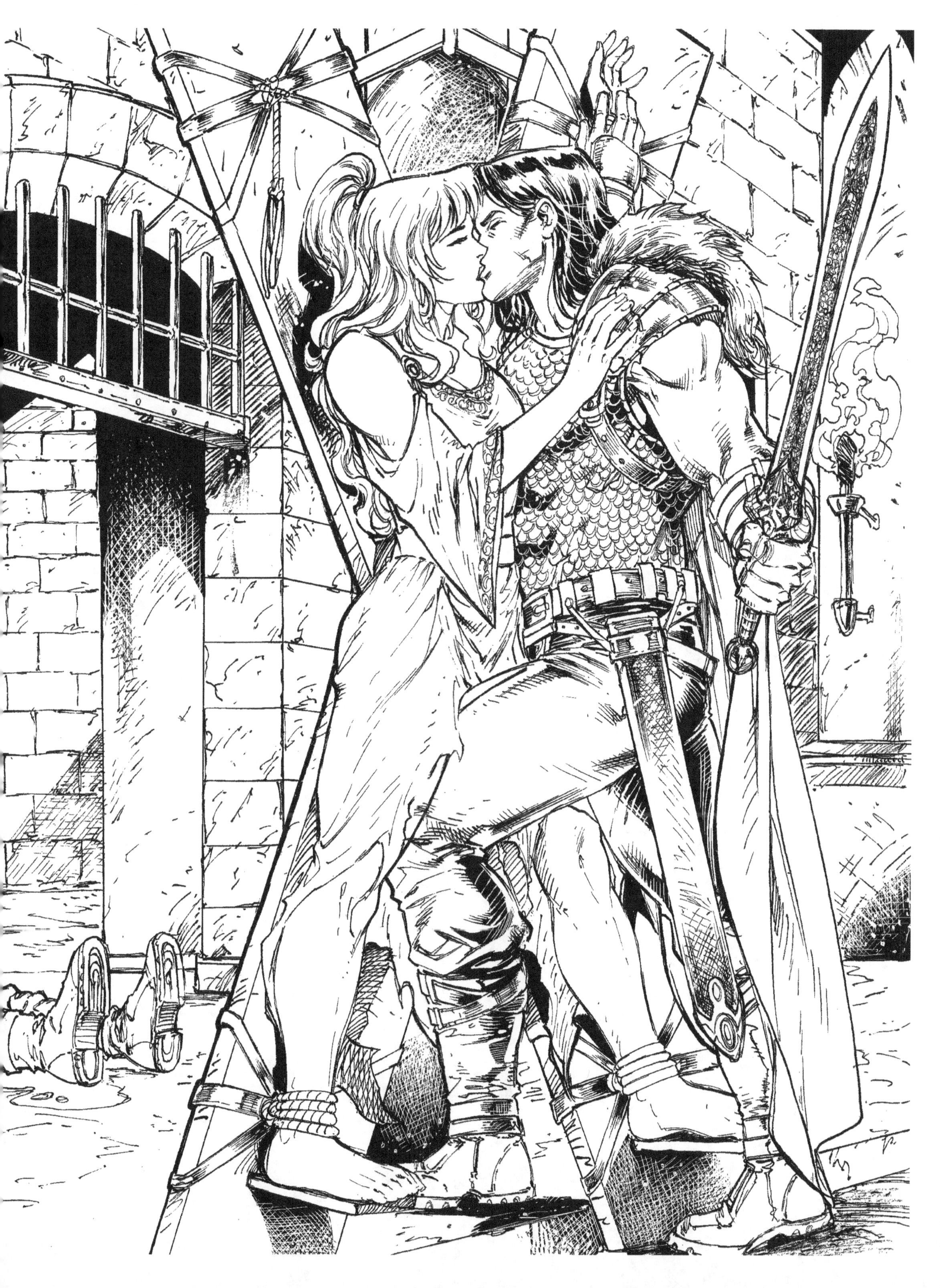

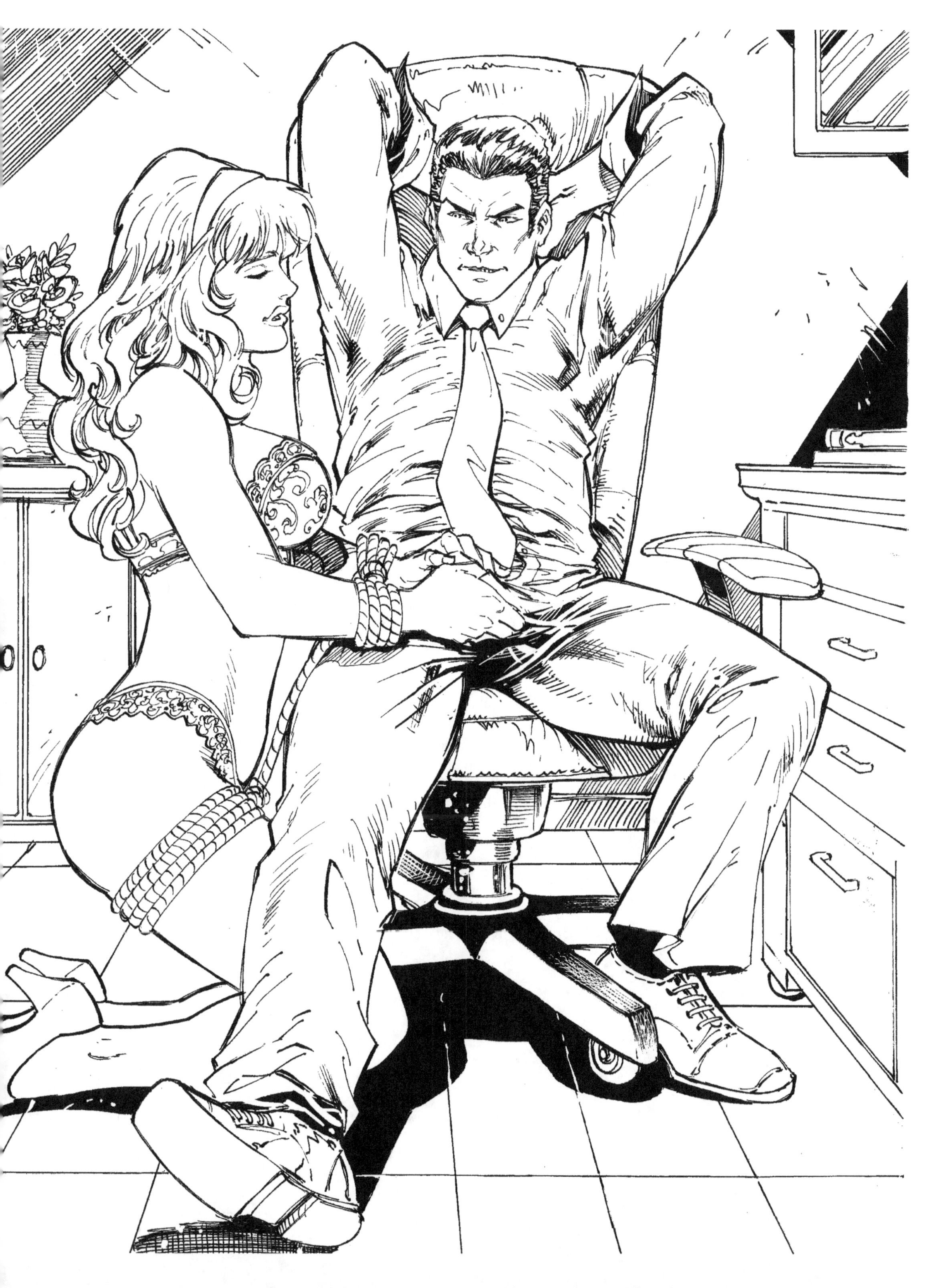

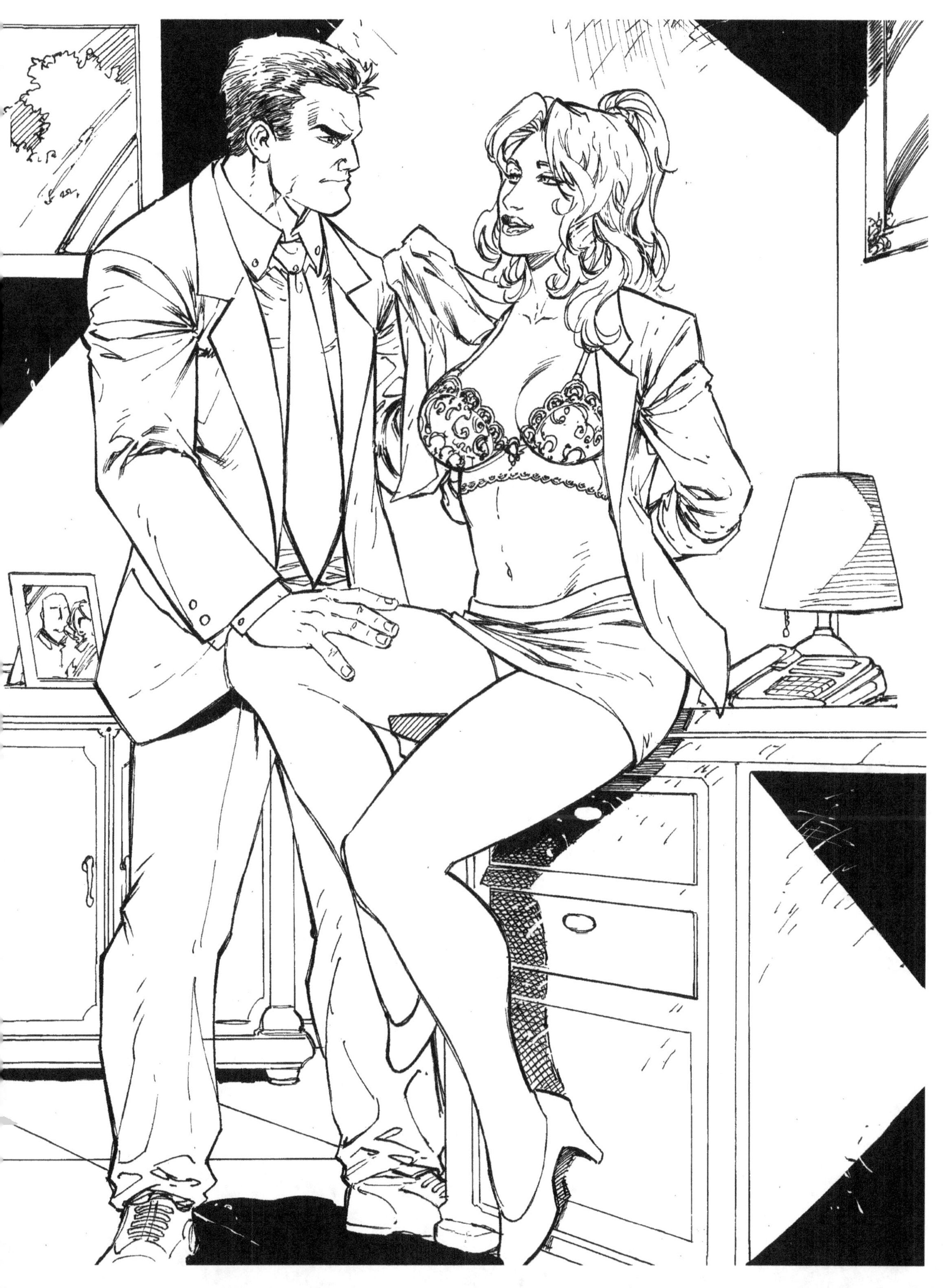

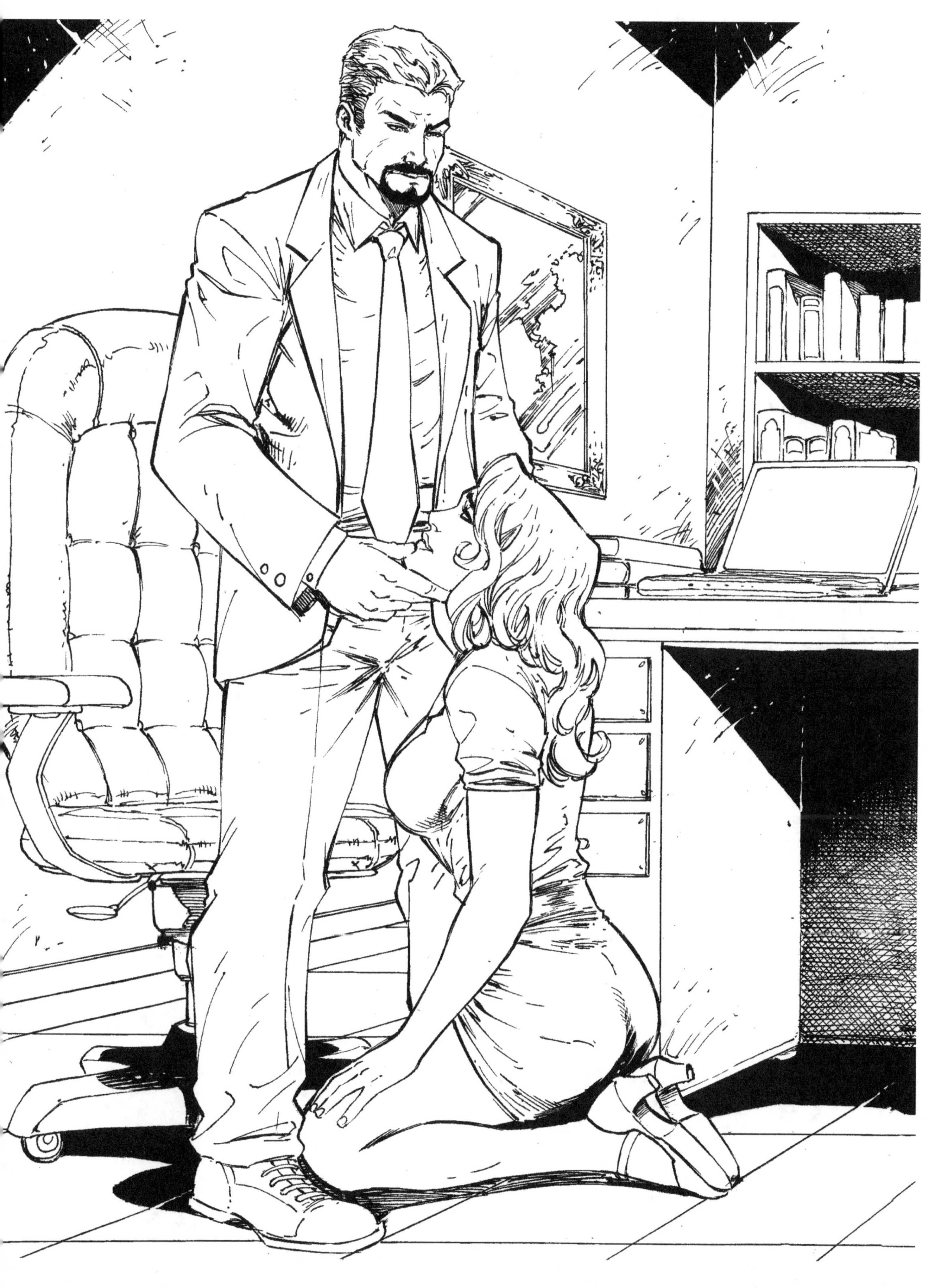

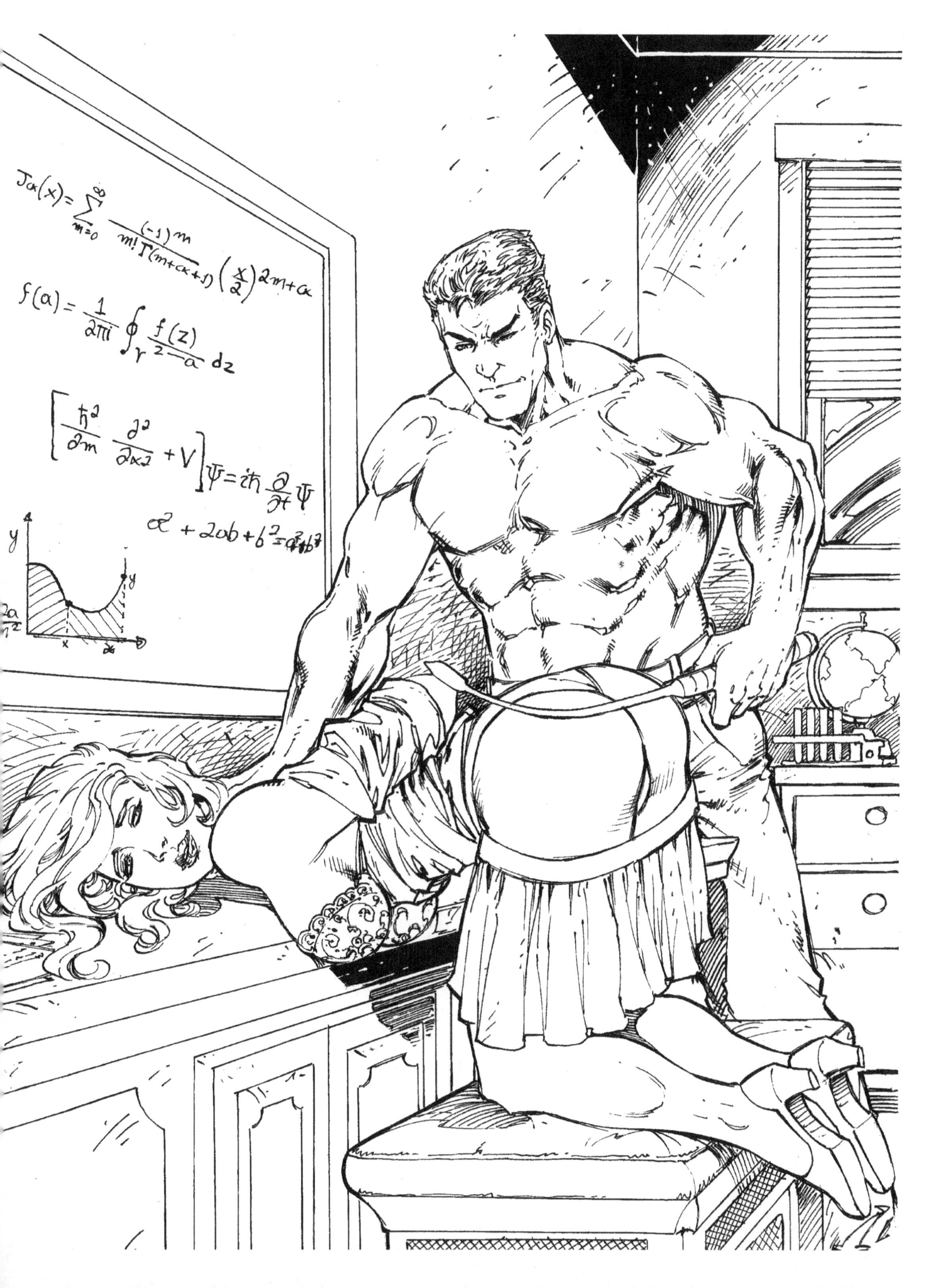

$J_\alpha(x) = \sum_{m=0}^{\infty} \frac{(-1)^m}{m!\,\Gamma(m+\alpha+1)} \left(\frac{x}{2}\right)^{2m+\alpha}$
$f(a) = \frac{1}{2\pi i} \oint_\Gamma \frac{f(z)}{z-a}\, dz$
$\left[\frac{\hbar^2}{2m} \frac{\partial^2}{\partial x^2} + V \right]\Psi = i\hbar \frac{\partial}{\partial t}\Psi$
$a^2 + 2ab + b^2 = a^2 + b^2$

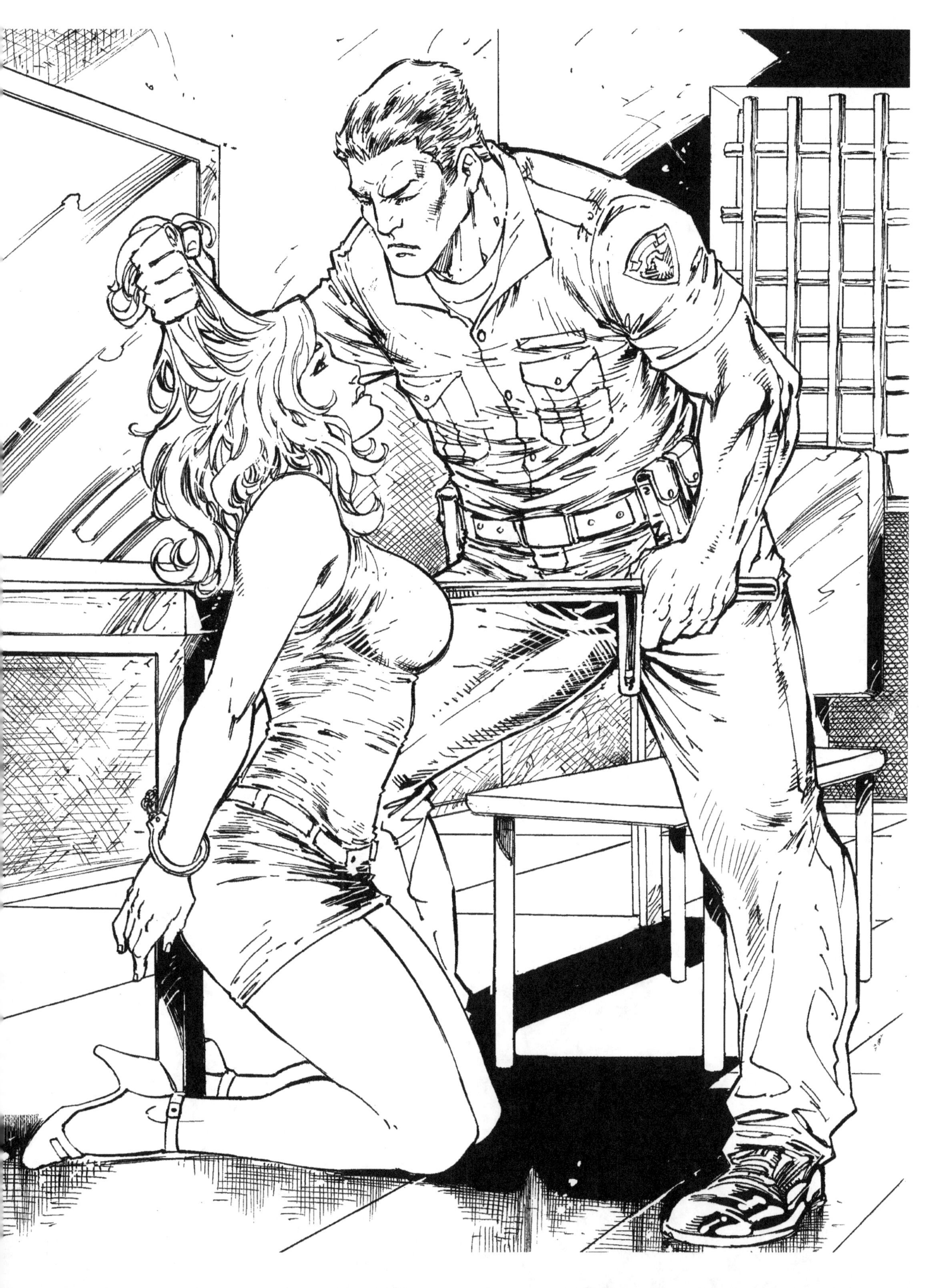

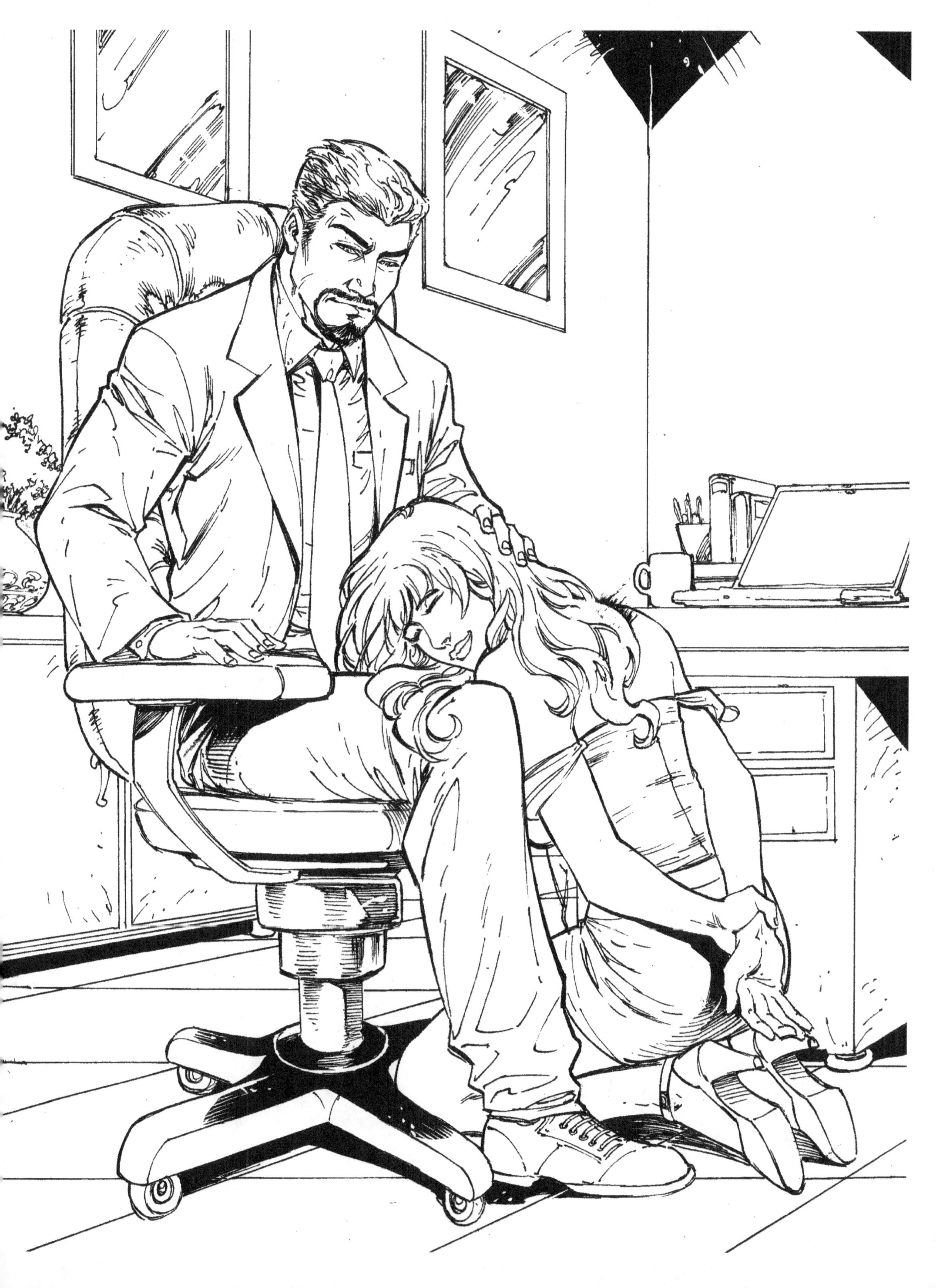

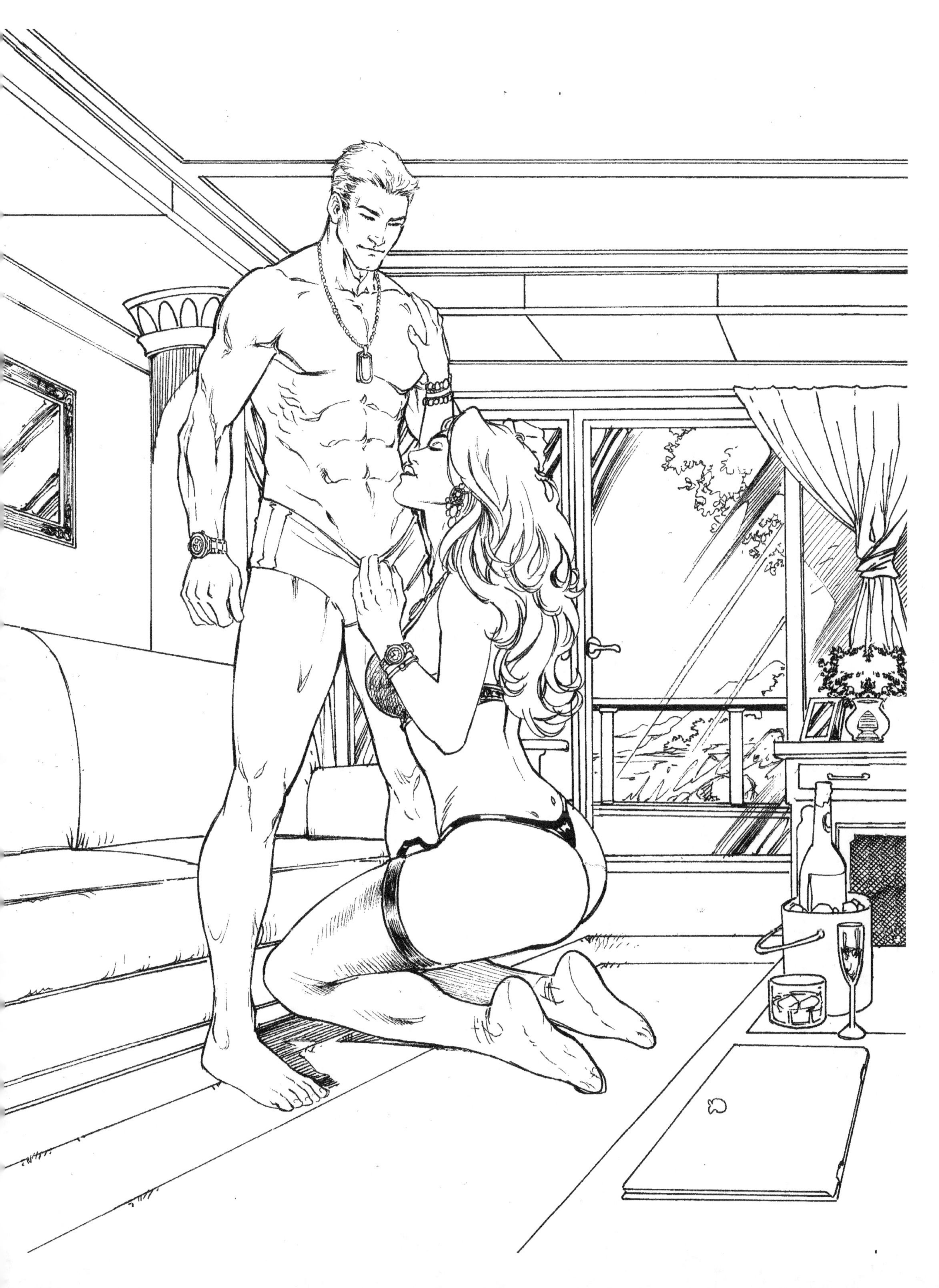

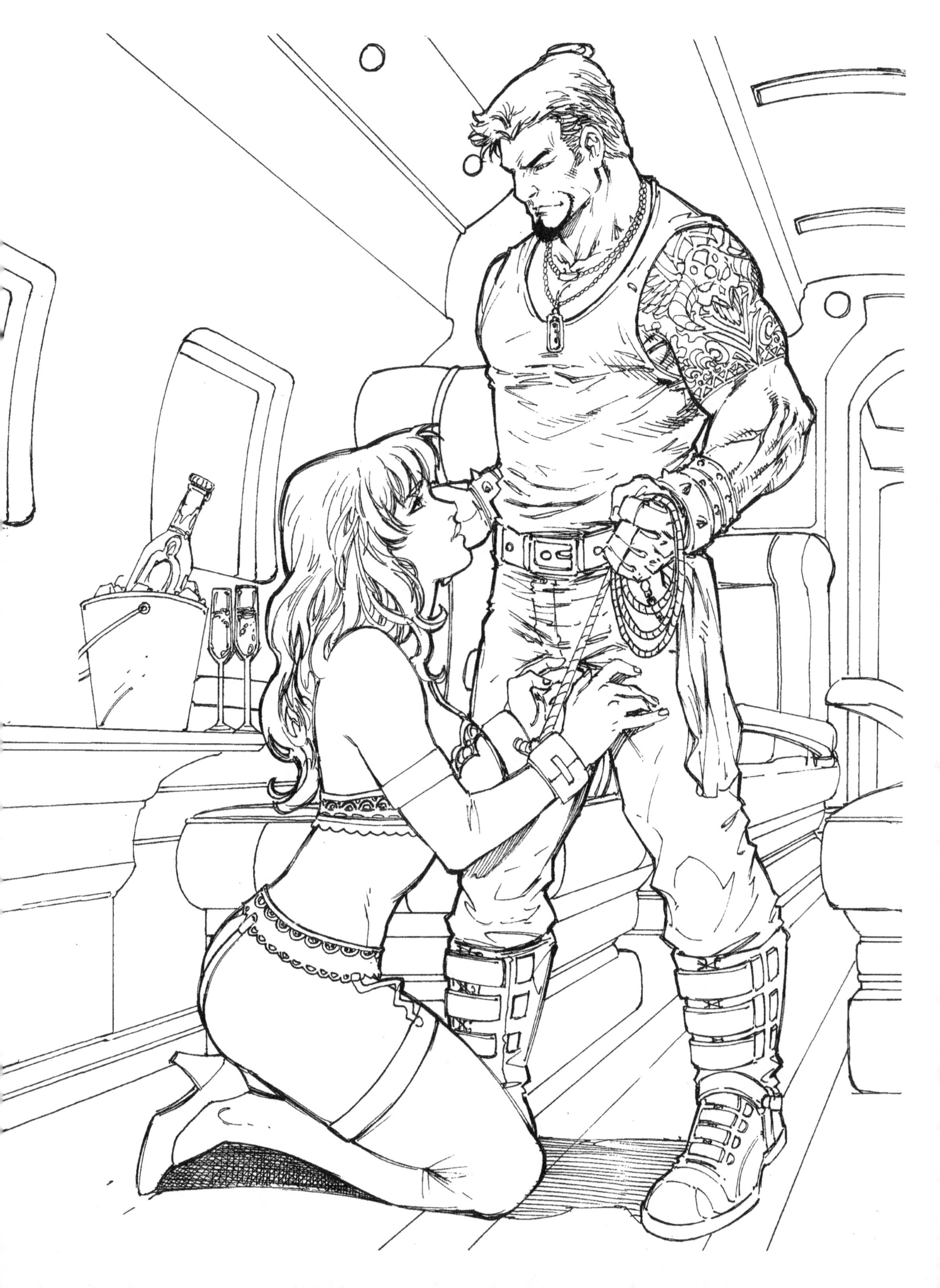

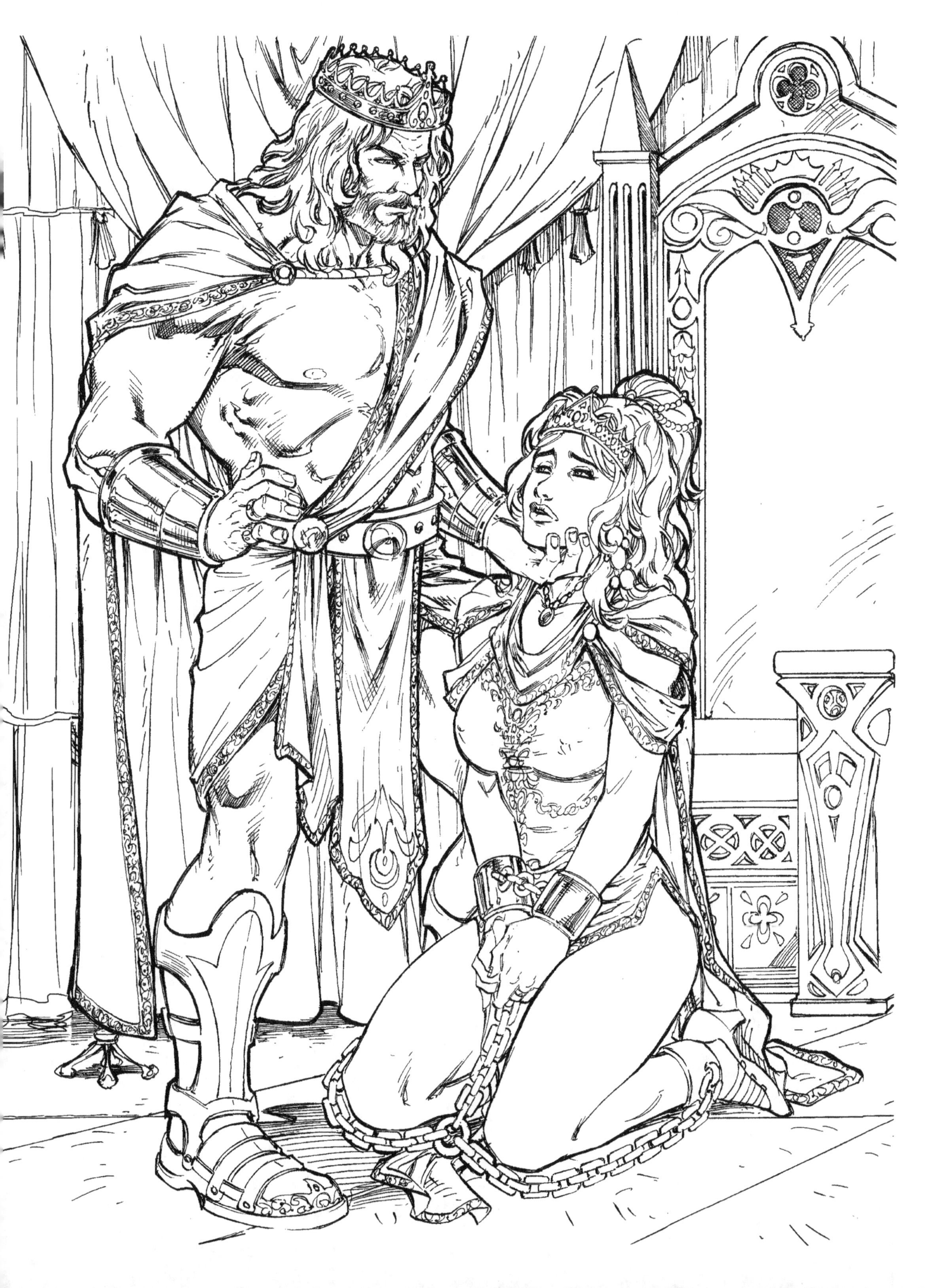

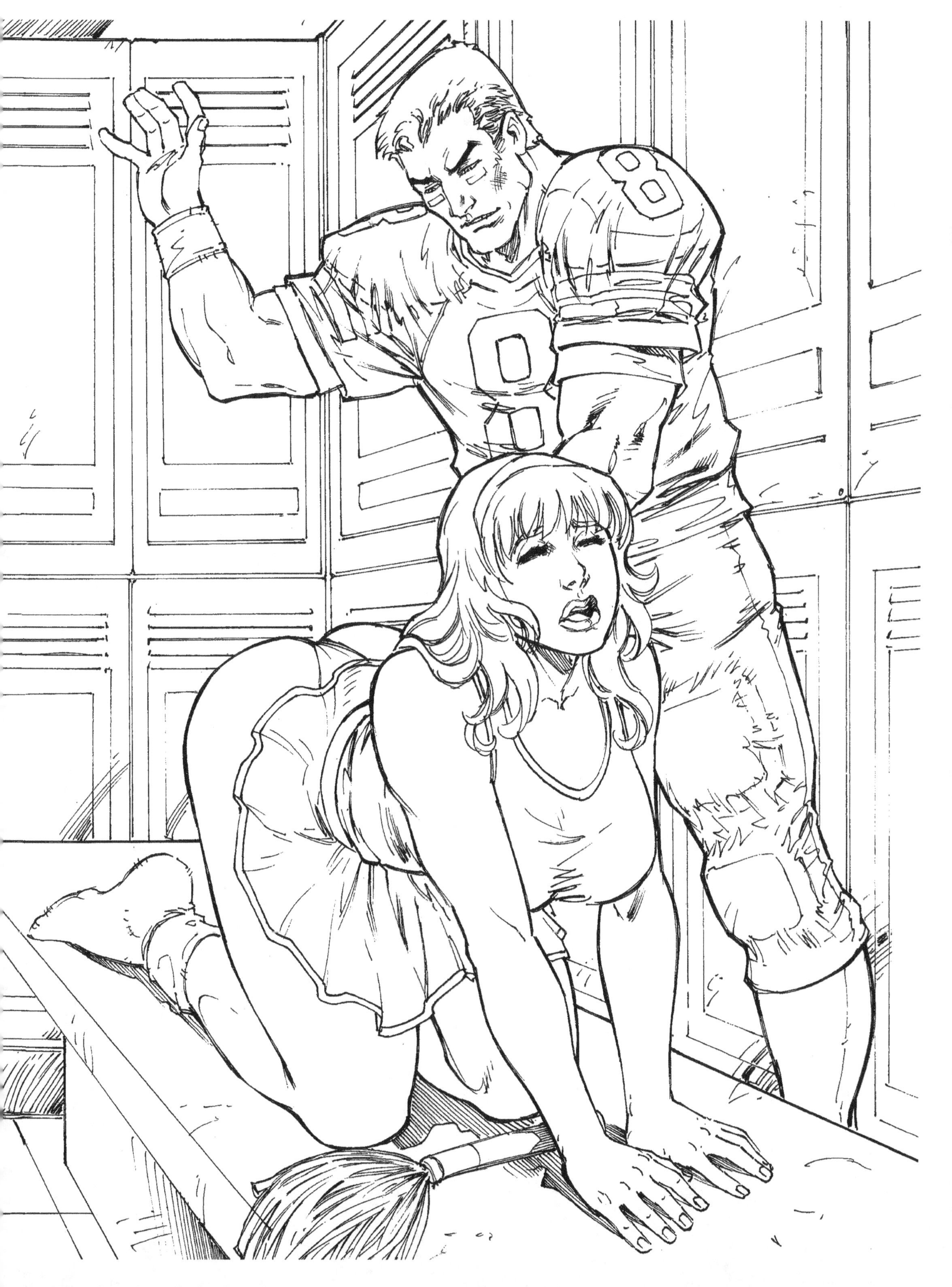

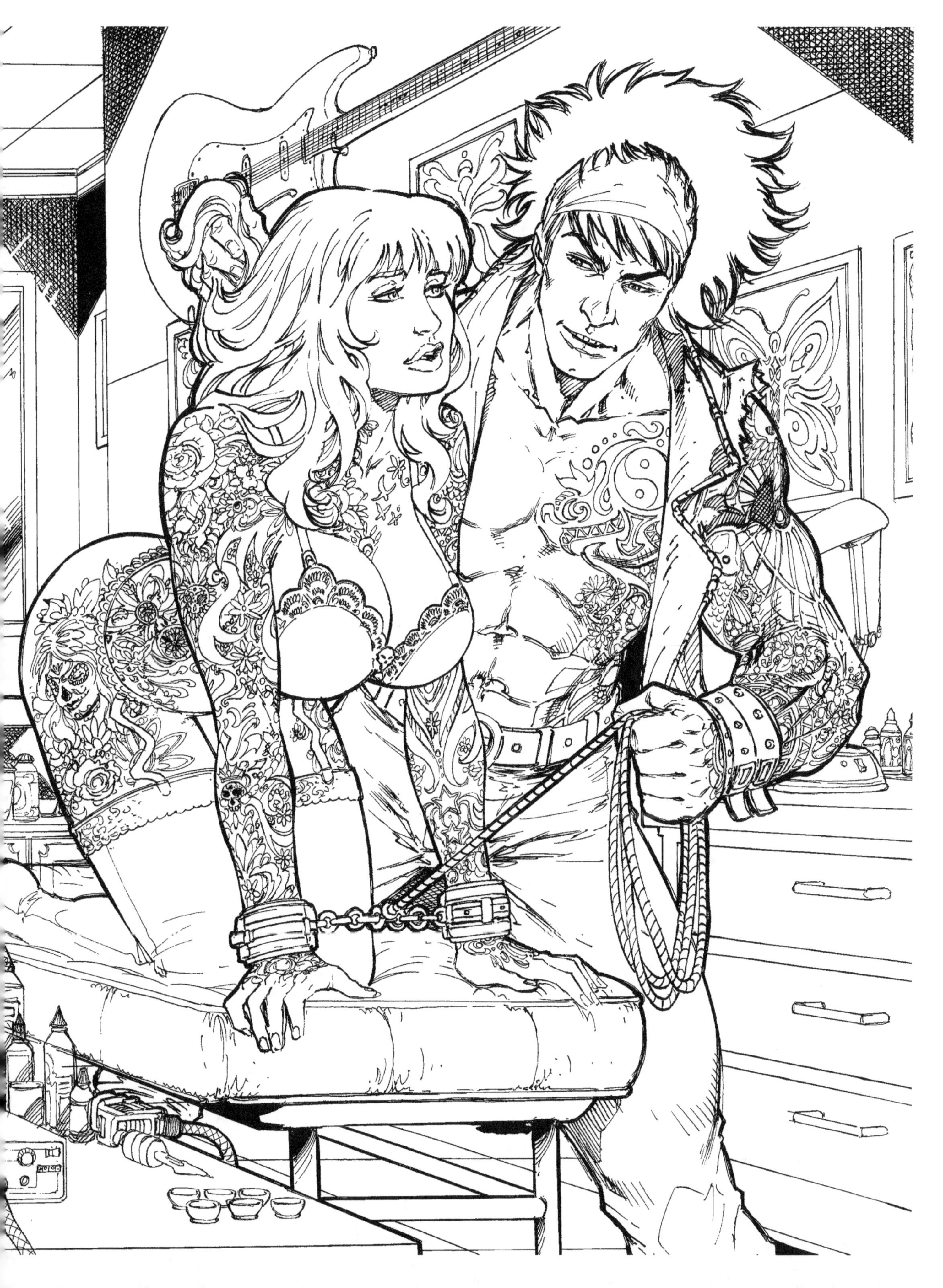

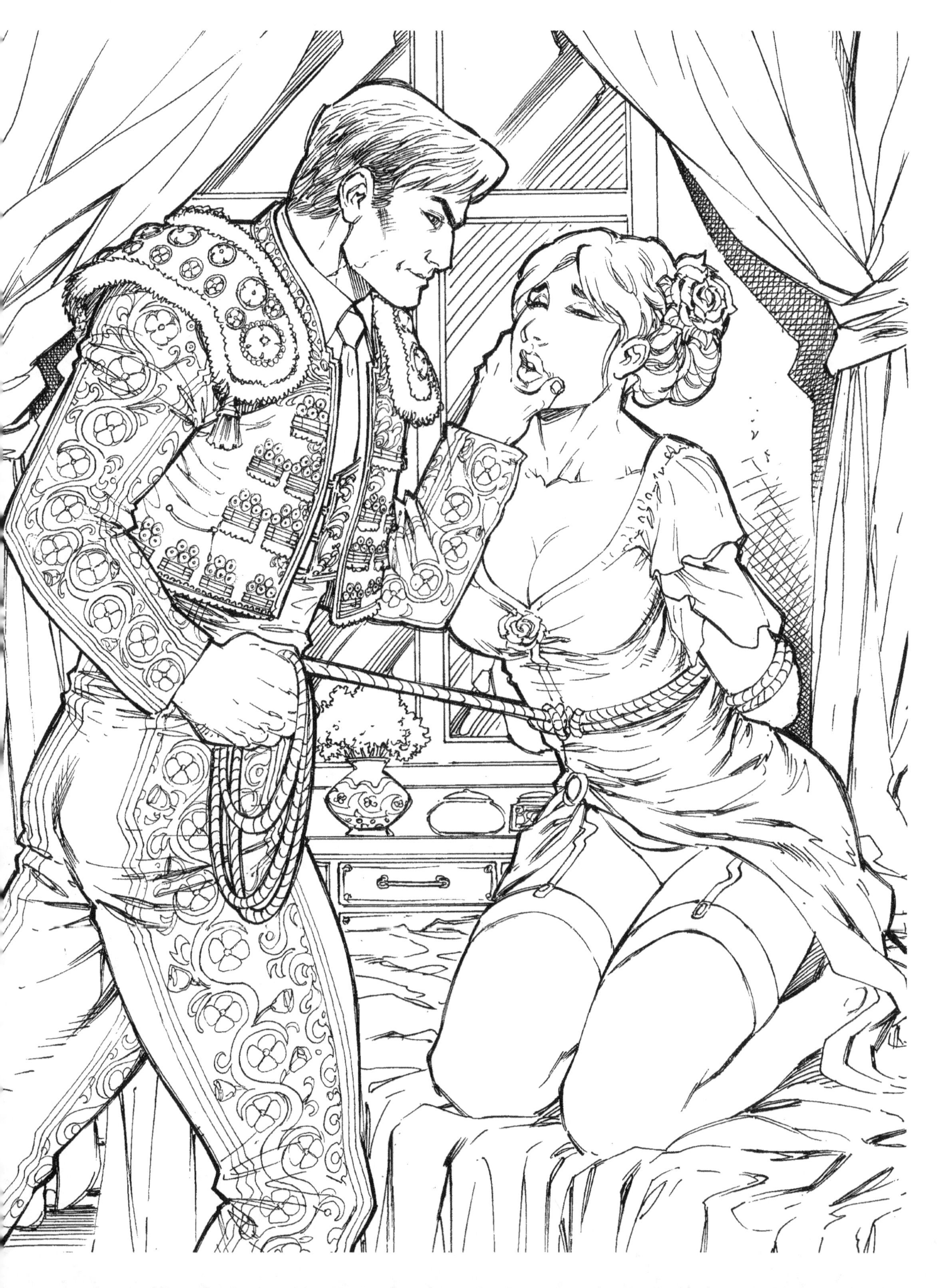

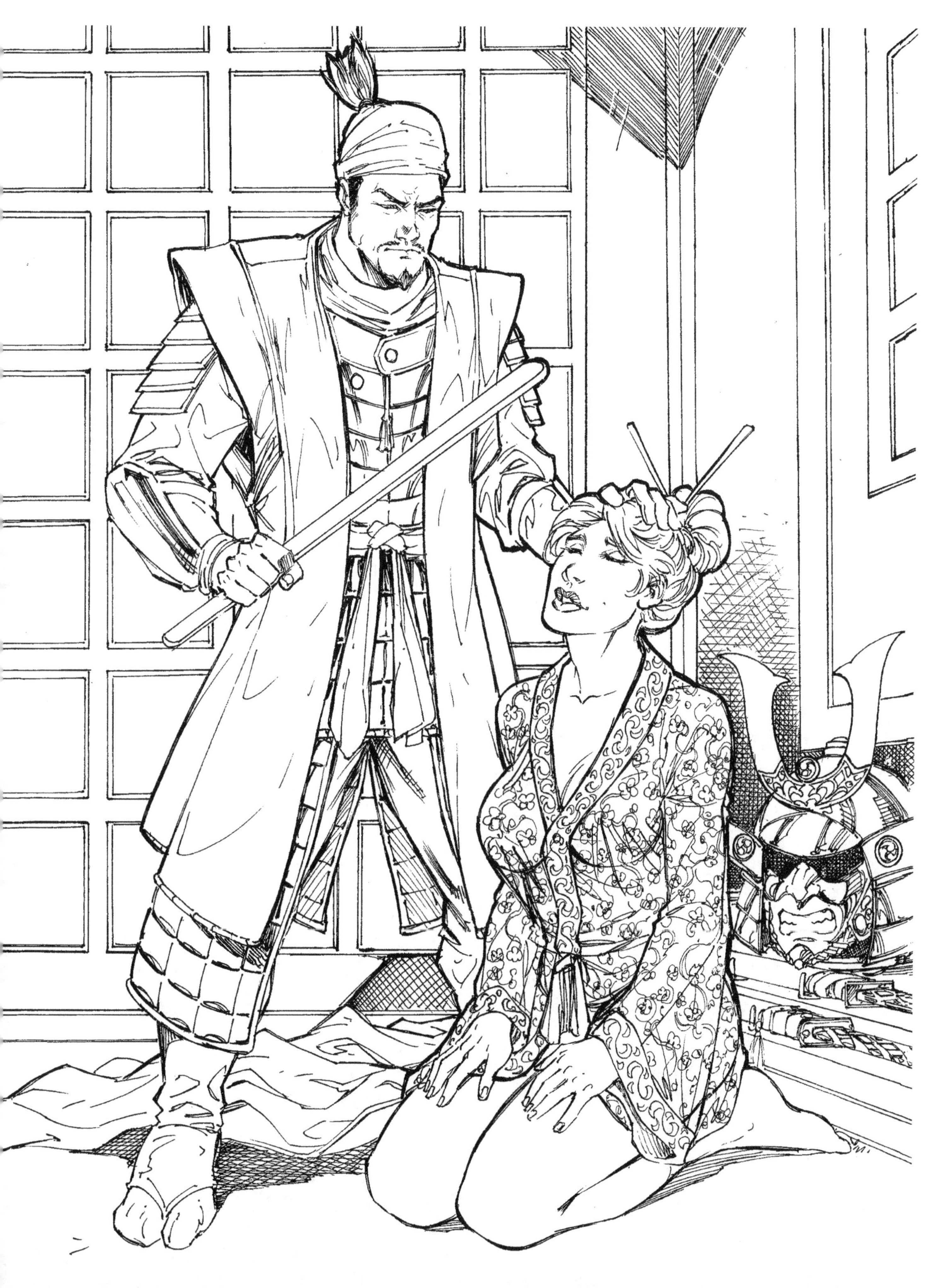

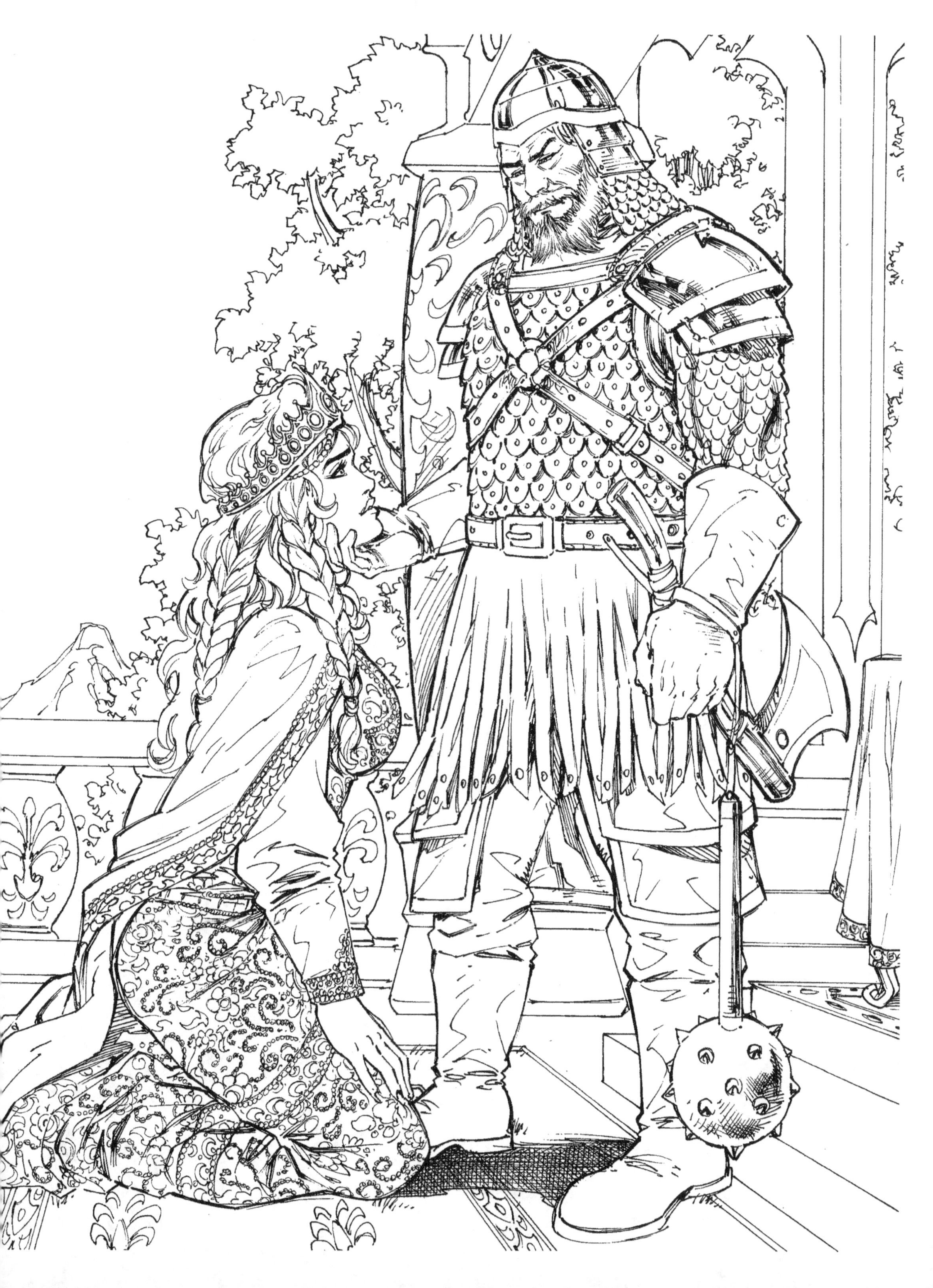

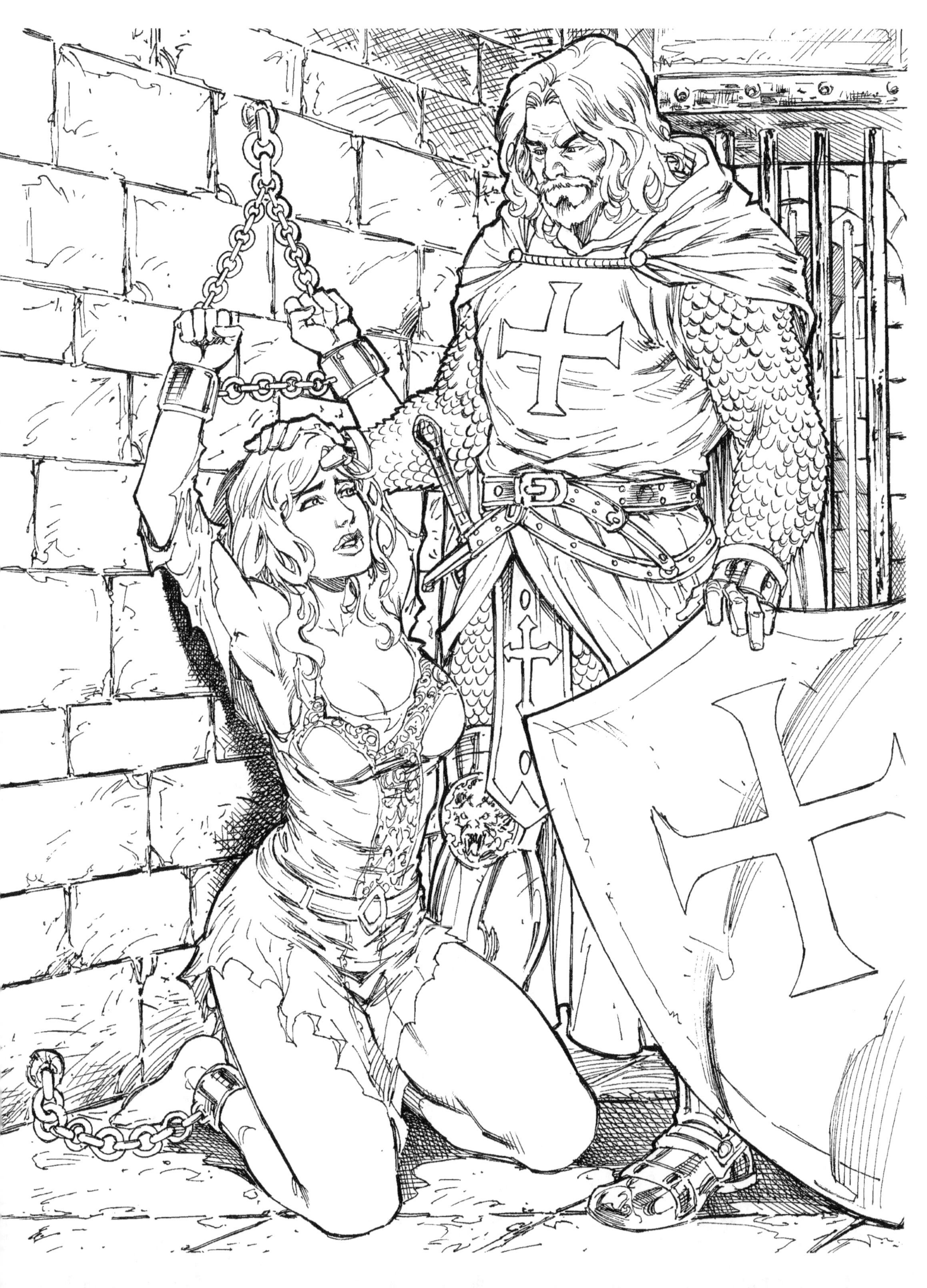

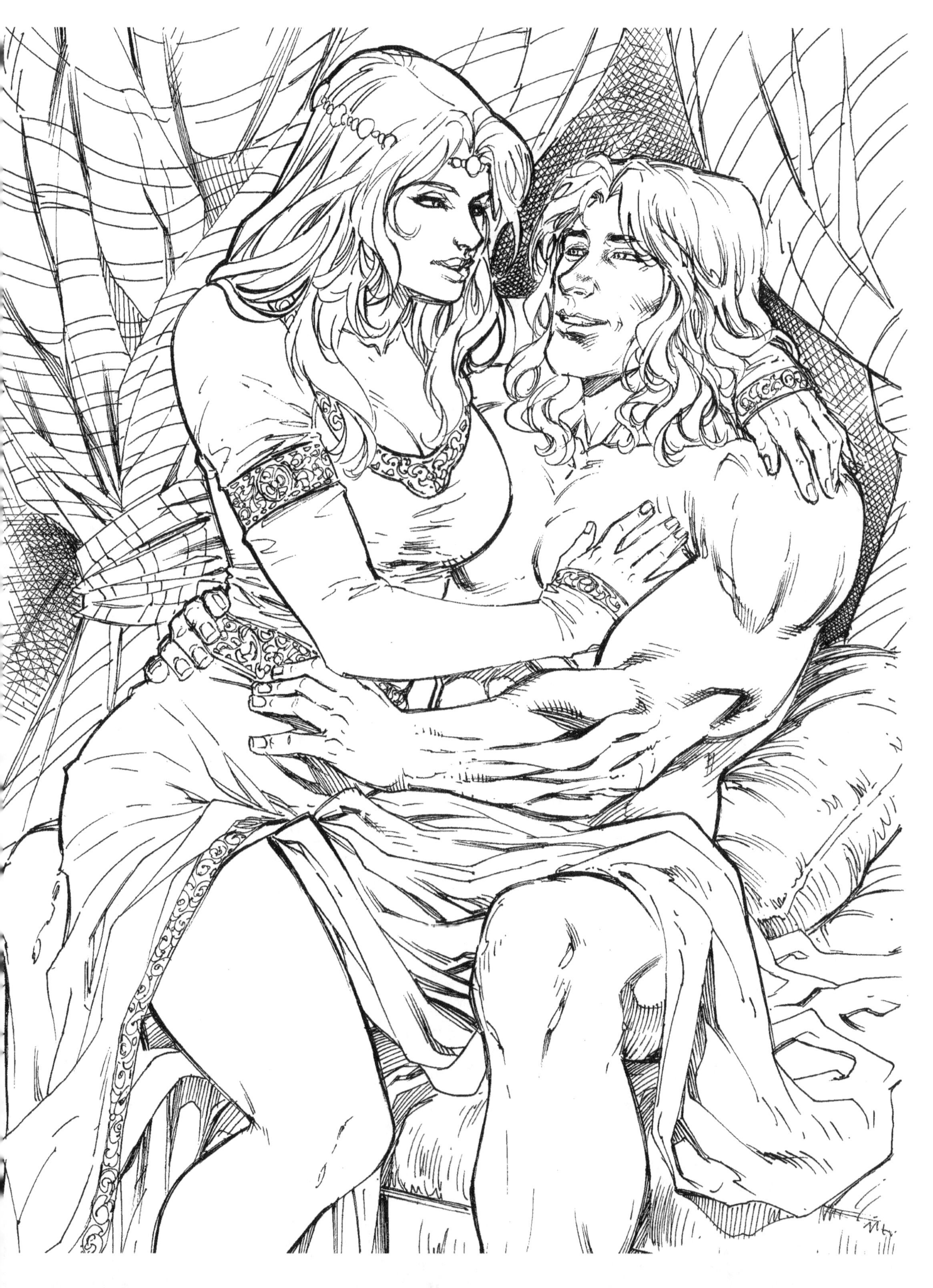

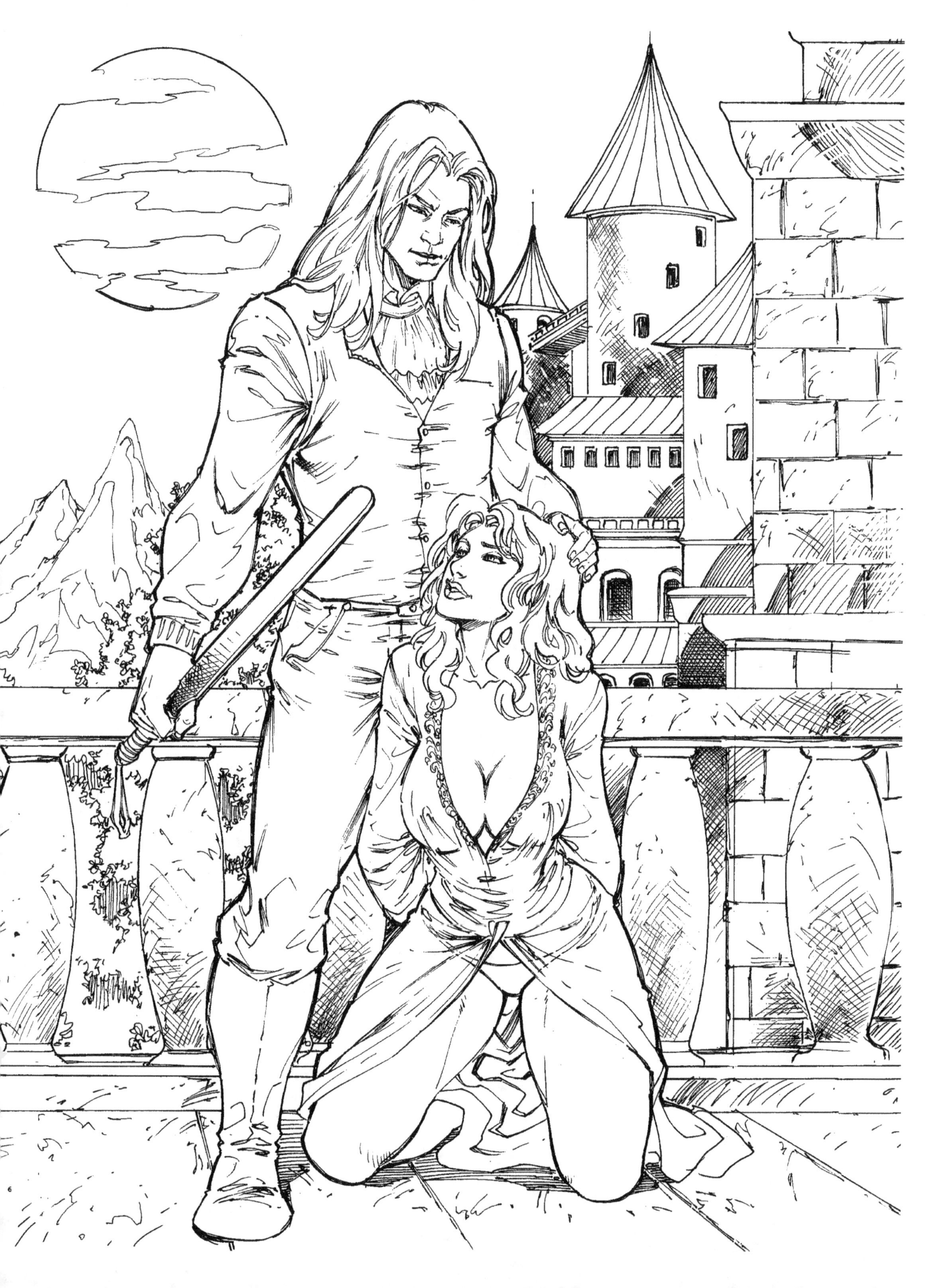

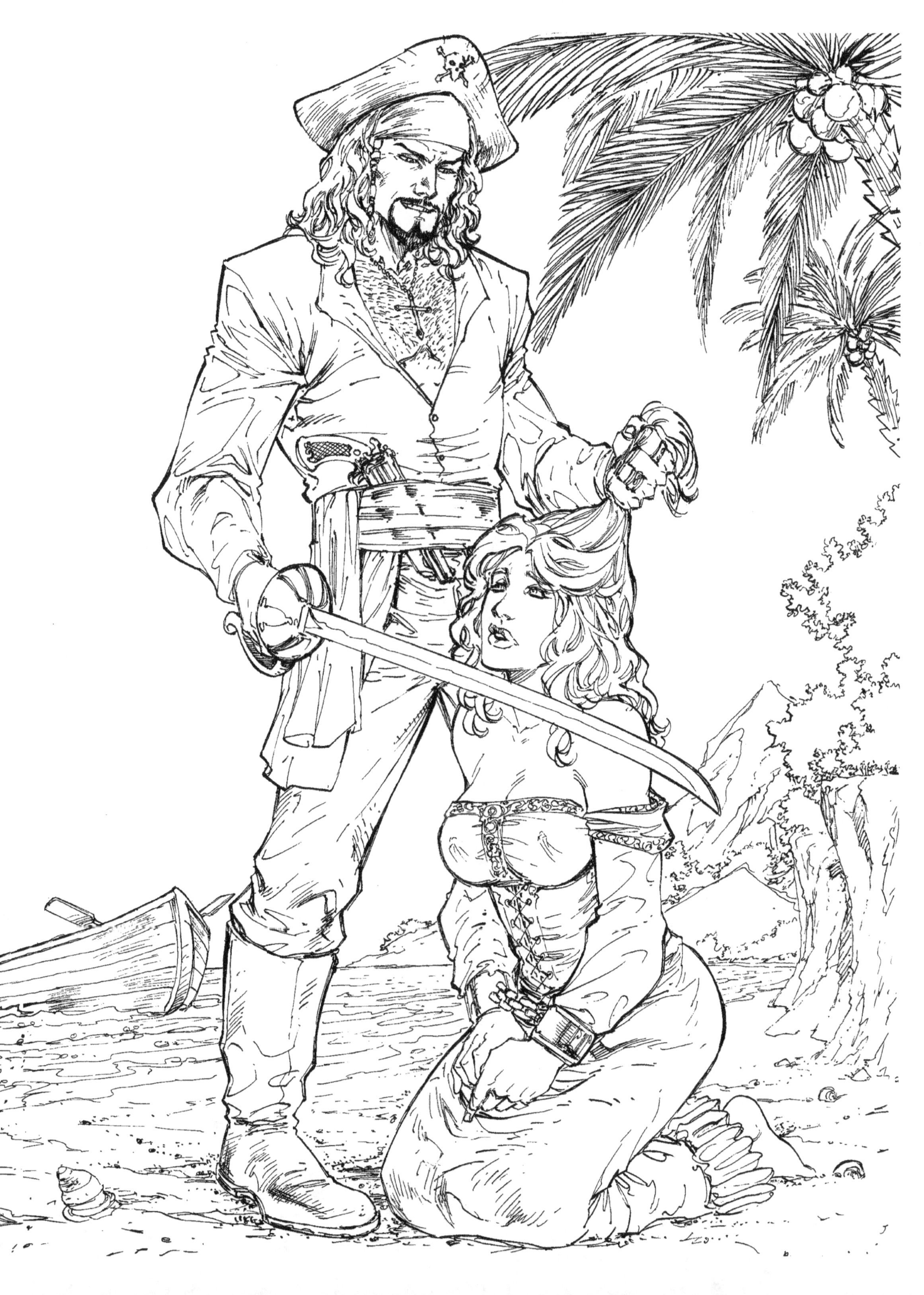

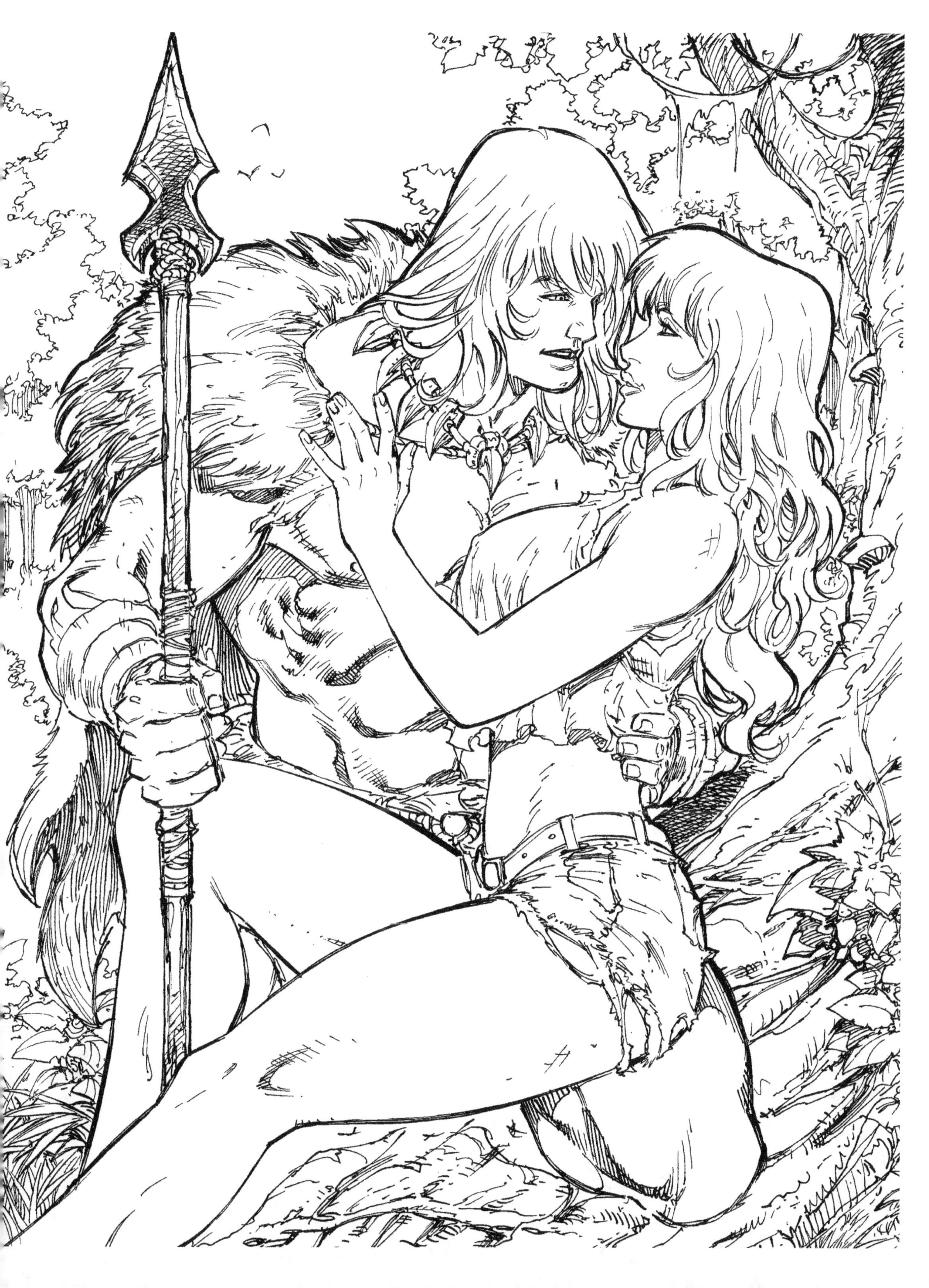

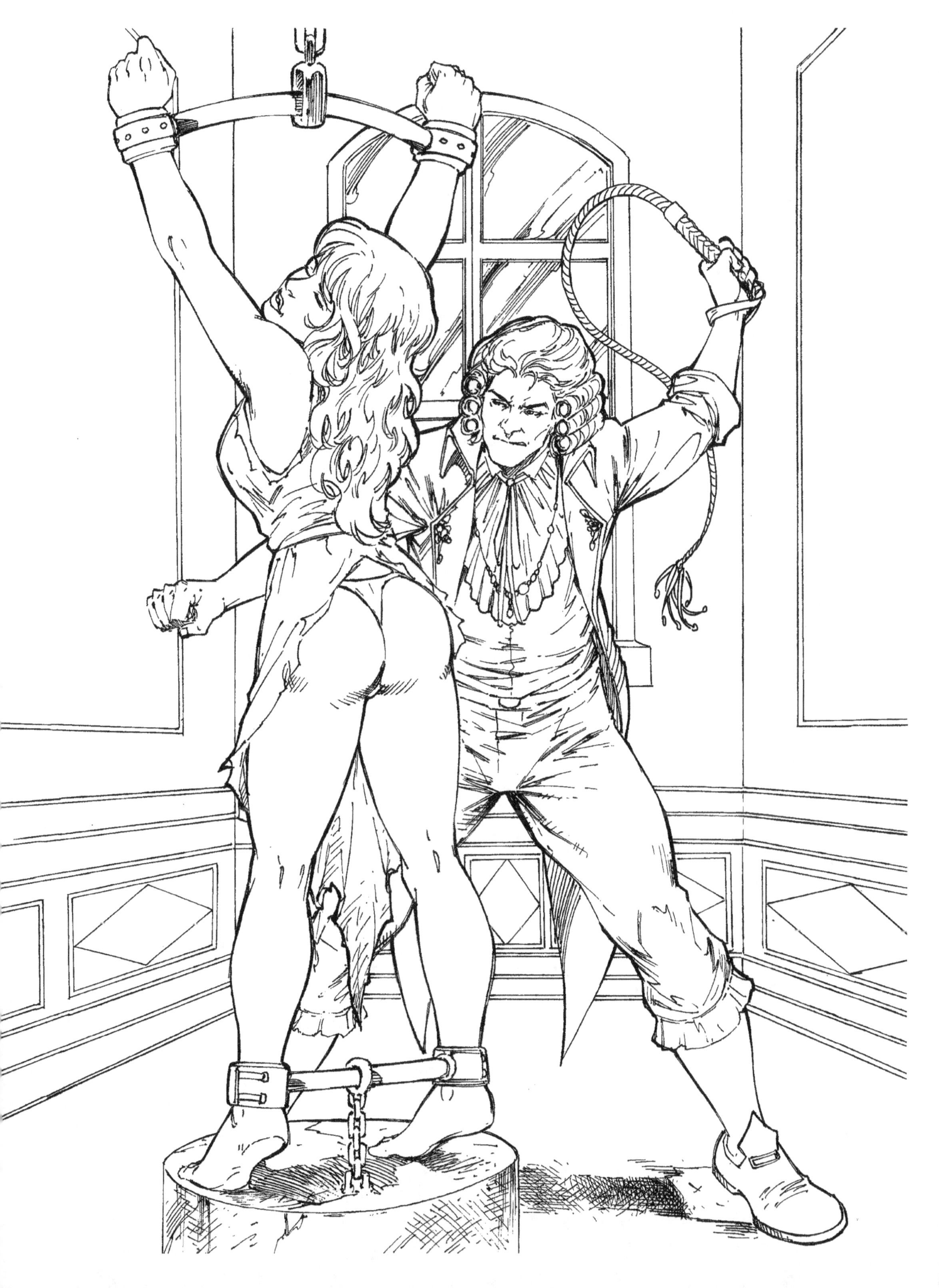

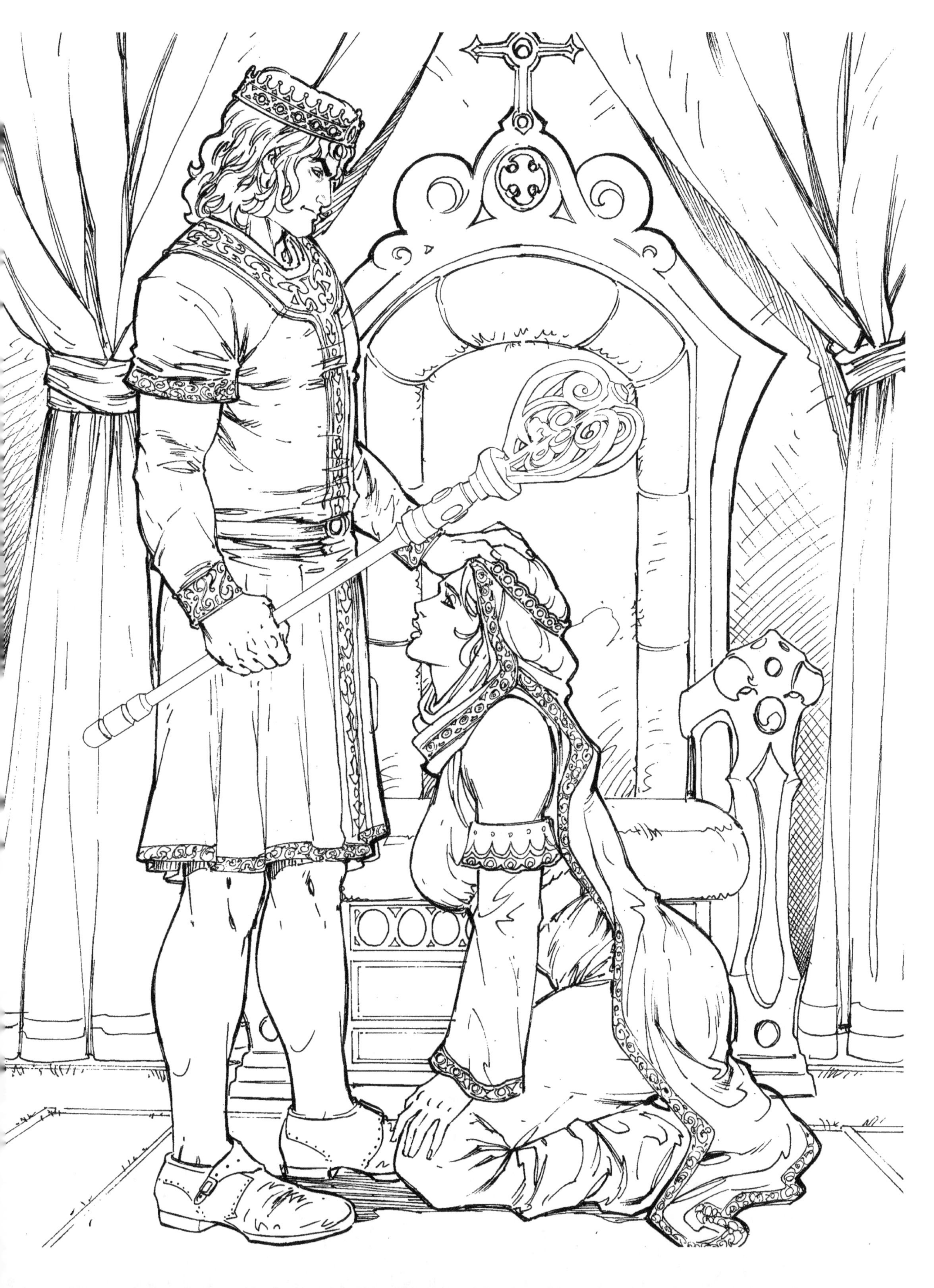

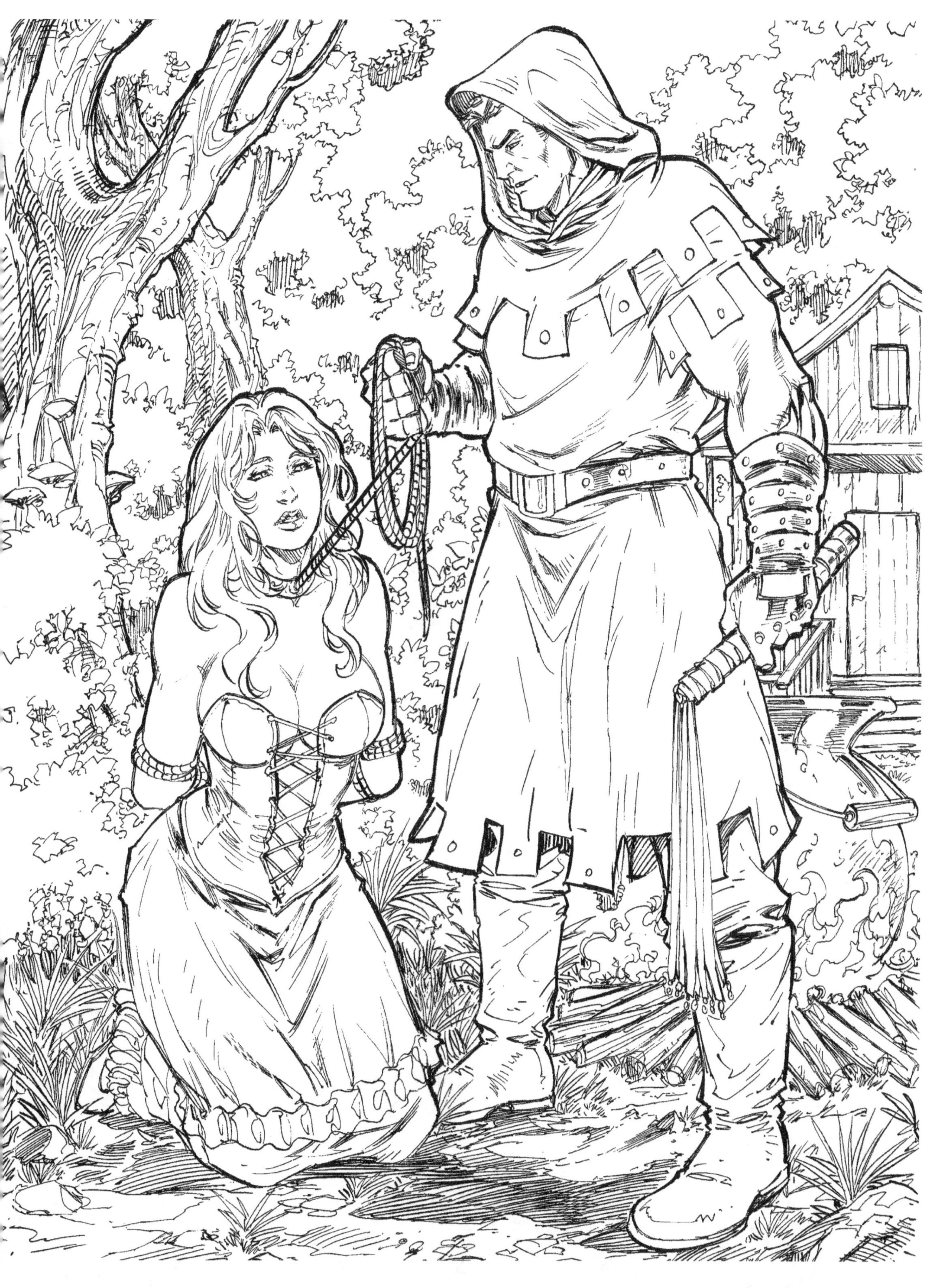

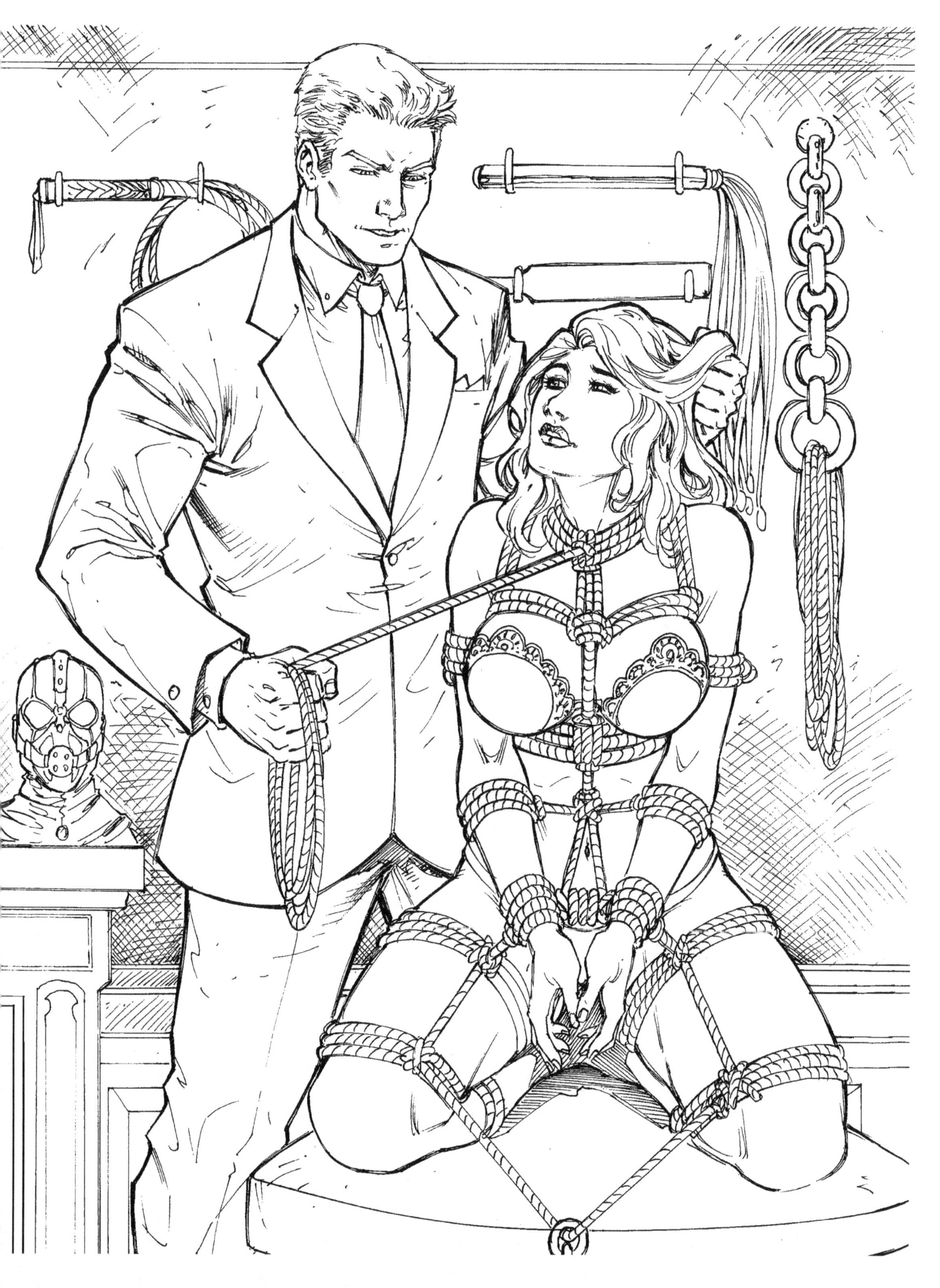

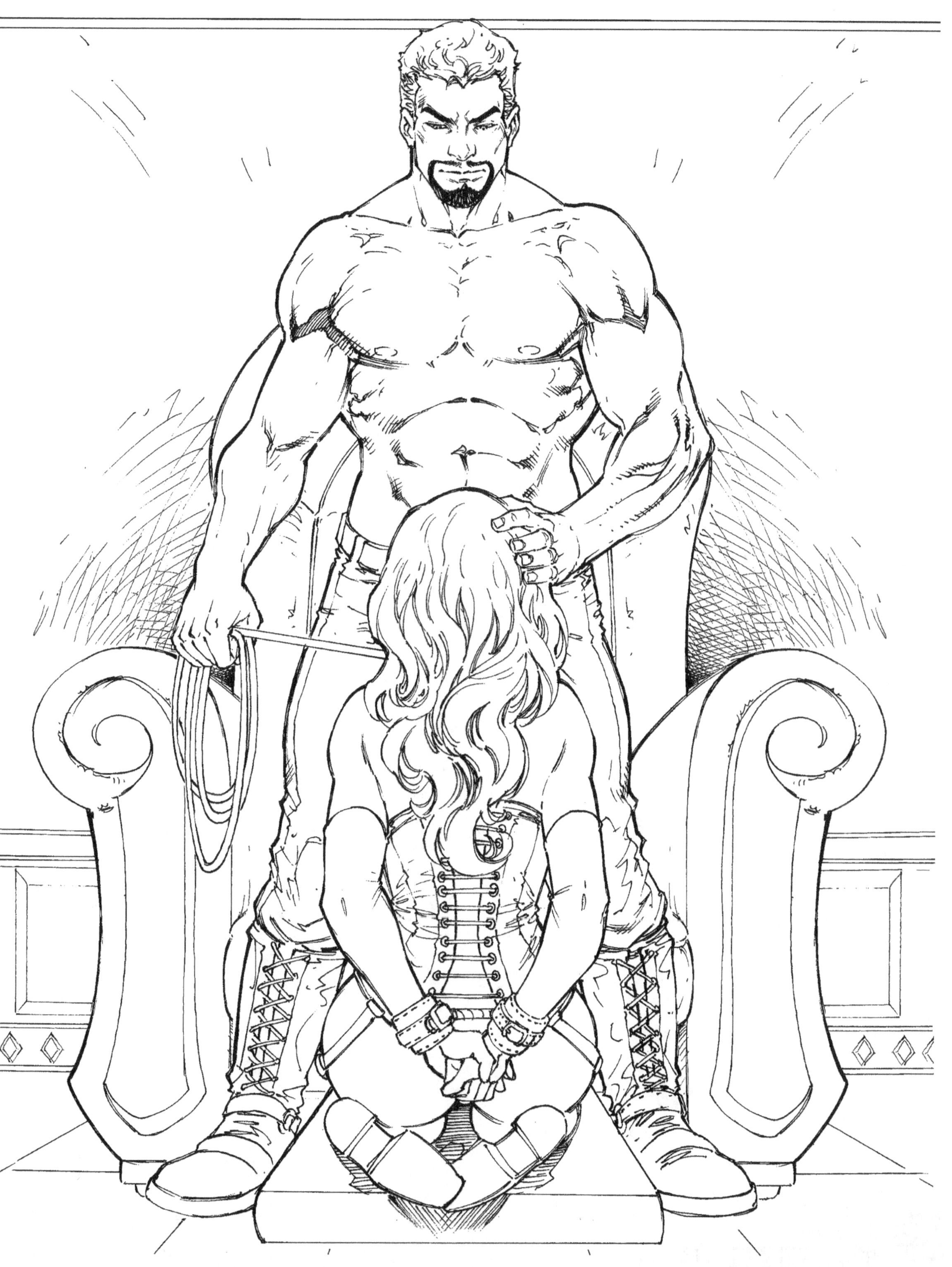